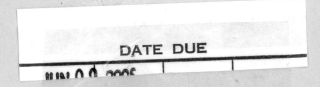
LOOK TEN YEARS YOUNGER WITHOUT SURGERY

THE BENEFITS.
THE RISKS.
THE SURPRISING DISCOVERIES.
THE AMAZING RESULTS.

*Learn the truth about Botox treatments and
how to make them work for you in*

THE BOTOX MIRACLE

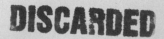

THE BOTOX MIRACLE

DEBORAH MITCHELL

Consulting Medical Editor:
ROBERTA D. SENGELMANN, MD

A Lynn Sonberg Book

POCKET BOOKS
New York   London   Toronto   Sydney   Singapore

An *Original* Publication of POCKET BOOKS

 POCKET BOOKS, a division of Simon & Schuster, Inc.
1230 Avenue of the Americas, New York, NY 10020

ISBN: 0-7434-6463-X

First Pocket Books trade paperback printing September 2002

10 9 8 7 6 5 4 3 2 1

POCKET and colophon are registered trademarks of
Simon & Schuster, Inc.

For information regarding special discounts for bulk purchases,
please contact Simon & Schuster Special Sales at 1-800-456-6798
or business@simonandschuster.com

This book is not intended to be a substitute for medical care and advice. You are advised to consult with your health care professional with regard to matters relating to your health, including matters which require diagnosis or medical attention. In particular, if you are taking or have been advised to take any medication, you should consult regularly with you physician.

Printed in the U.S.A.

ACKNOWLEDGMENTS

My sincere thanks to Roberta Sengelmann, MD, for her expert and enthusiastic guidance during the production of this book. She was always there when I needed her. I also thank Leslie Baumann, MD; Robert N. Butler, MD; Ronald Fragen, MD; Ghazala Hayat, MD; Debra Jaliman, MD; Gary Monheit, MD; and John F. Romano, MD, for their helpful contributions.

CONTENTS

FOREWORD

Now is a great time to be aging. That may sound like an odd thing to say, but the truth is, today we are much better equipped to fight the signs of aging than we were, say, ten years ago. We have at our fingertips many wonderful, proven ways to improve the appearance of our skin. New advances in cosmetic enhancement and skin rejuvenation are being introduced all the time. We have techniques and products that allow us to move into maturity gracefully without changing who we are, without requiring a lot of downtime, and without causing a lot of troublesome side effects and risks. And now we have an exciting, innovative addition to the skin enhancement scene that meets all those requirements—Botox injections.

It's true that Botox has been used for cosmetic purposes for about ten years, even though during much of that time most of the general public didn't know about it. Yet with the recent approval of botulinum toxin A (Botox) by the Food and Drug Administration (FDA) for treatment of frown lines, the drug has been catapulted into the media and into the minds of mainstream America. Suddenly, people everywhere are talking about Botox. More and more physicians in cosmetically oriented fields are being trained in the proper use of Botox and are advertising their new skill. Unfortunately, inadequately trained personnel at health spas and salons who may have little to no medical background have also jumped on the Botox bandwagon. Men and women are being invited to Botox "parties." They are being told that getting Botox is "no big deal."

But it can be a big deal: it's a medical procedure, it involves injecting a potent neurotoxin into your facial muscles, and it can give you some very positive and pleasing results. It's a big enough deal that if you are considering Botox injections, you should stop and ask questions of yourself and your doctor before you undergo treatments. I believe that when you decide to pursue a cosmetic procedure, you should take the time to make sure you have all the facts before taking the plunge. This is the simplest way to avoid untoward side effects.

This book can answer those questions for you. It can help you decide if you are a candidate for Botox. It introduces you to the pros and cons of getting the injections, a history of the drug, how treatments work, and what happens during a typical injection session. It helps you find the best qualified doctor for your treatments and talks about other cosmetic procedures that you may or may not choose to complement your Botox injections. It even discusses the medical uses of Botox, such as treatment for crossed eyes and migraines. And, because aging gracefully is about more than eliminating wrinkles, it also explores ways to keep your skin healthy, through nutrition and supplements, and which ingredients in your skin care products really do what they claim to do.

In my work as director of the Center for Dermatologic

and Cosmetic Surgery at Washington University School of Medicine in St. Louis, I have been using Botox increasingly over the past six years to where now, I administer Botox injections almost daily. I have been heartened by the positive responses from the people I have treated. People come to me saying, "I don't want to look different. I just want to look better and more rested." After they get their injections, they are thrilled with the results. They like what they see when they look in the mirror. It's wonderful to help improve people's quality of life.

I think it's important and valuable that how we look and how we feel be in sync. Yet many people feel out of sync. They feel a lot better than they think they look. When they stand in front of the mirror, they see frown and scowl lines, crow's-feet, and bags under their eyes. What they see on the outside doesn't reflect how they feel inside.

Although we can't wipe away all traces of maturity and aging, even with all the advances in cosmetic dermatology and surgery, I don't think that's the point. The point is not to stop aging but to age smoothly, gracefully, and with style. We now have ways to improve people's appearance without downtime, big risks, and great expense.

Although some people still have to justify for themselves why they want to look beautiful or handsome, I believe such thinking is becoming obsolete. While some people may think it's vanity that makes men and women want to improve their appearance, I have some people come to me and say, "I'm not especially vain, I just want to look better." I tell them it's okay to want to look as good as you feel. You should not feel guilty because you want to look attractive, optimistic, and happy. We've gotten past passing moral judgment on ourselves for dyeing our hair to keep the gray away, so why should we neglect our skin and let it age without grace?

It's very confusing for the general public to figure out what is good and what is not good for their skin, which doctor is best qualified to do a particular procedure, and whether a specific procedure is even a reasonable option for them. When they read something in a men's or women's magazine, they think it's the truth. It's difficult to separate the hype from the science, especially when companies use a few catchy phrases like "wrinkle reduction," "antioxidants," and "replaces what your skin has lost" to lure consumers and suddenly everyone is marketing the same products.

I'm a firm believer in education and in the concept that knowledge is power. I also consider myself to be a patient advocate, and I want people to do what works best for them. This book offers readers information they can use to help them make decisions about their skin rejuvenation that will give them the results they desire.

In the rapidly changing world of cosmetic skin enhancement, it's important to keep up with the new products and procedures and what they can and cannot do for you. Botox injections are just one dramatic example of the positive changes taking place in cosmetic dermatology, and I think it's important for people to learn all they can before they take that step. I hope everyone who reads this book walks away with a greater understanding of Botox and a better appreciation for all they are and all they can be.

Roberta D. Sengelmann, MD, Director
Center for Dermatologic and Cosmetic Surgery
Washington University School of Medicine, St. Louis

1

THE PROMISE OF BOTOX

THERE'S NO DENYING IT: the anti-aging revolution is here, and looks matter. More specifically, looking young . . . or younger . . . matters. Even though we know that everyone ages, and that science has yet to find a way to stop the physical signs of the march of time, there *are* ways we can reduce the wrinkling, sagging, and loss of radiance that go with it.

Studies prove that how we feel about our appearance can have a tremendous impact on self-esteem and self-confidence, and as a result, it can affect virtually every aspect of our lives—from success on the job to success in our love lives. But you probably don't need researchers with clipboards to convince you of this.

Ingrid is a good example. At forty-three, she has kept her slim, athletic figure from her early twenties, and she's a bundle of energy. When she was thirty-eight, after her two children were in school, she went back to college and got her degree in business management. Now she works at a stock brokerage and wants to go on and get her broker's license. Yet something is holding her back.

"Inside I feel like I'm twenty-one," she says, "but on the outside, well, that's a different story." She points to the furrow between her brows and the crow's-feet around her eyes. "The up-and-coming brokers in my office, and in the field for that matter, are young. Or at least they look young. So I believe I need to look as young as I feel in order to be a successful broker."

She frowns, emphasizing the lines that are causing her so much anxiety. "I know getting rid of these wrinkles won't make me perfect, but I'm not looking for perfection. But I do believe eliminating them will make a big difference in my career and in how confident I feel about my abilities as a broker. And so I've decided to do something about them."

HOW BOTOX CAN HELP

Ingrid is certainly not alone. Every year in the United States, millions of men and women undergo one or more cosmetic procedures that in some way enhance or change their appearance. From chemical peels to nose reconstruction to eyelid tucks, dermatologists, plastic surgeons, and other cosmetic surgeons across the country are reshaping the way Americans look, and as a result, how they feel about themselves.

Now we have another cosmetic procedure to add to the list, an important new tool—approved by the Food and Drug Administration (FDA) in April 2002—in our quest to look and feel younger: Botox Cosmetic (referred to after this point simply as Botox).

Injections of Botox, one of the fastest-growing cosmetic procedures on the market today, are used for the reduction or elimination of facial wrinkles caused by dynamic, or hyper-functional, muscles (muscles that get a lot of use). Those are the wrinkles that form when you contract your facial muscles to form a frown, squint, grimace, smile, or other type of ex-pression, resulting in those tell-tale lines around your eyes, mouth, or nose, and across your forehead. Botox can be very effective in temporarily getting rid of some, but not all, of your facial wrinkles. But before we talk about which wrin-kles Botox can banish, let's find out more about this popular substance.

WHAT IS BOTOX?

Quite simply, Botox is a type of toxin produced by the bac-terium *Clostridium botulinum*. If you're thinking that some-thing sounds familiar about this substance, that's because this bacterium is the same one that causes botulism, or food poi-soning. It's also the same bacterium that some countries stockpile as a bacterial weapon. You might be wondering if this is a substance you would want injected into your face.

Thanks to the wonders of medical technology, injecting Botox into the face isn't only possible, it's being done thou-sands of times a day, and safely. In the late 1970s, scientists discovered that botulinum toxin, when it was diluted to a great degree, had some very positive characteristics, proper-ties that could bring significant relief to thousands of people who had specific neuromuscular problems throughout the body. (We'll talk more about those medical uses later, in chapter 5.) And after years of science and serendipity, experts discovered that botulinum toxin A (the bacterium has eight different toxins, or serotypes, each named for a letter of the alphabet) has cosmetic uses as well, especially when it comes to getting rid of wrinkles in the upper third of the face—that is, along the forehead and at the outer corners of the eyes.

If you're familiar with the concept of homeopathy, you'll see a similarity with Botox. In homeopathy, a substance—sometimes one that is poisonous when taken at regular strength, such as arsenic—is diluted to such a tremendous degree that when it is finally ingested, it is completely safe. Botulinum toxin is extremely potent, but Botox injections contain a greatly diluted form of the toxin, rendering the injection safe yet effective.

THE DESIRE TO LOOK YOUNG

Own up to it: you may believe the old adage that wrinkles add character to a face . . . but you don't want it to be *your* face, at least not just now when you're thirty or forty or fifty. You, like Ingrid, want to look as young as you feel. And why shouldn't you?

The desire to look young and beautiful is far from new. Since ancient times, both men and women have searched for ways and concocted formulas to look more youthful. Eye and face cosmetics were used by the ancient Egyptians, the most famous of whom is Cleopatra, who was known to use lactic acid to peel her skin to look more beautiful. Archaeologists have found formulas, written on papyrus, that explain how to prepare mixtures of plants and honey for women to use as facials. Archaeological digs have also uncovered many containers that once held green malachite, black antimony powder, and lead sulfide, all types of minerals that were ground up and used as cosmetics.

Ancient people even performed crude cosmetic procedures to improve—in their opinion—people's appearance. In western Russia, for example, a broad, flat nose was considered beautiful, so parents would bind the nose of a child to achieve this result. Because the Chinese believed that dainty feet were a sign of wealth and beauty, the practice of binding the feet of girls to prevent foot growth existed for thousands of years. Among some African tribes, an elongated neck is considered a thing of beauty, so some women keep adding rings around their necks to gradually stretch it to a desirable length.

Modern-Day Cosmetic Procedures

As we've seen, there have always been people who are willing to undergo different procedures or use various products to help them look young and beautiful. Apparently many people still feel similarly. According to the American Academy of Cosmetic Surgery, 623,588 Botox procedures were performed in 1999, two years before the Food and Drug Administration (FDA) even approved Botox injections for cosmetic use. These procedures, which were done to reduce or eliminate wrinkles on various sites on the face and neck, are known as "off-label" uses (once a drug has been approved for one use, it can legally and ethically be used for other purposes, at the discretion of the practitioner). Botox has been approved for various medical (that is, noncosmetic) uses since 1989. And its off-label uses for cosmetic purposes continue to grow: in 2000, the number of procedures was 730,787; in 2001, it ballooned to 913,484.

FDA-Approved for Cosmetic Use

With the new FDA approval of Botox on April 15, 2002, for removal of frown lines—also known as glabellar lines—on the forehead, experts believe the number of procedures will greatly surpass the million mark. Right now, only one other cosmetic procedure—chemical peels—is performed more often: more than two million people undergo them each year. And some combine a chemical peel with Botox injections to get rid of wrinkles and improve skin texture.

It's important to note that **the only cosmetic use the FDA has approved Botox for is the removal of glabellar lines.** However, doctors have been using Botox for cosmetic reasons in this and other areas of the face for about ten years. Some of the wrinkle sites, like smile lines that run from the nose to the corners of the mouth and down the sides of the mouth, do not respond as well to Botox because the facial lines that form there are not as strongly muscle-driven as those in the other regions. However, Botox can be used along with other cosmetic procedures to get the look you desire. We will talk about some of those options in chapter 9.

But overall, the risks of Botox, when administered by a knowledgeable professional, have been very low. And this safety factor has fueled a growing interest in Botox among people of all ages.

Who Is Getting Botox Injections?

Botox injections have become all the rage, and not just among aging baby boomers. Approximately 17 percent of the people who underwent Botox injections in 2000 were between the ages of nineteen and thirty-four, hardly an age group one usually associates with bothersome wrinkles and aging skin problems. By far the largest percentage of Botox users was the 35 to 50 age group, at 41 percent. Those in the 51 to 64 age group counted for 29 percent, with men and women 65-plus rounding out the total at 13 percent.

Did we say men? Yes, as of spring 2001, about 12 percent of those getting Botox injections were men. And the number of men seeking Botox injections is expected to grow.

"We do a lot of men," says Ronald Fragen, MD, of Fragen Cosmetic Surgery Center in Palm Springs, California. "I think about 50 percent of men pay attention to their looks. For them, Botox is an easy, convenient way to accomplish the look they want."

And it's not just actors, jet-setters, and chief executive officers who are lining up for their injections. Dr. Fragen reports that construction workers, police officers, social workers, and others from all walks of life are looking to get rid of their wrinkles.

Why is everyone doing it? If you're like Ingrid, you may want to look younger to help advance your career. Robert, a fifty-two-year-old computer salesman, felt the pressure from his younger colleagues as he traveled around the country and attended conferences and sales conventions. "No one said anything to my face, but the general feeling I was getting was, it's a young and vital industry, and you'd better look young and vital to stay in the game."

With layoffs happening all around him, Robert decided he needed to get rid of the frown lines that pocketed his forehead and the crow's-feet around his eyes, and to lift his sagging eyelids. The procedures took years off his face, he says, while adding years to his career.

"Now I feel I can compete with the so-called younger guys," he says with a smile that leaves his forehead wrinkle-free. "I've got a family to support, two kids going to college, and I need to stay in my high-paying field. I consider the doctor's fees to be a small investment in my face, and one that will pay off big in the long run."

Or, you may just want to feel better about yourself. Nedra had just ended a three-year relationship with Tom, after she caught him with another, younger woman. "I was devastated," she said, "and the fact that he left me for someone younger—she's twenty-five, I'm thirty-four, and Tom's thirty-five—really got me thinking. Did I look old? Did I act old? I took a good look in the mirror and decided that time wasn't being kind to my face. All those years on the beach had taken their toll, and the wrinkles were creeping in. The frown lines were very noticeable, yet I hadn't noticed them while I was with Tom."

Now, sans Tom, she made an appointment with a dermatologist, who explained the various options for removing wrinkles. One of those options was Botox injections to remove her forehead wrinkles.

"The whole idea of Botox appealed to me," she said. "I like the idea that it's fast and essentially painless. I can go on my lunch break and be right back at work in about an hour."

Nedra kept her first Botox injection appointment and then waited for results. "In less than a week I was looking great!" she said. "I just love the results. My friends can't believe the difference in me, not only in how I look, but in my attitude as well. I feel so much younger. Removing those wrinkles gave me such confidence. I'm *not* old, and now I don't look old. Botox did that for me. It's the best decision I ever made."

Is Botox Safe?

Fast, easy, painless, and you'll look younger. What more could you ask for? That's why Botox injections seem like a good decision if you want to get rid of frown lines quickly.

And while it sounds like it may be the answer to your desire to eliminate wrinkles, it's not a decision you should make lightly or without considering all the facts, options, and possible complications. After all, Botox *is* a drug, and one of the most toxic substances in the world. True, what you receive via injection is a greatly diluted version of the toxin, and Botox has been shown to be very safe. However, side effects are possible with even the most benign substances, and Botox is no exception. And because you will be accepting treatment into an area of your body, you want to make sure you are aware of all the possible complications, as well as all the benefits, of getting Botox injections.

That's why we wrote this book: to help you decide whether Botox is right for you, and if it is, how to make sure you get the most expert treatment available. As you go through this book, you will also discover that Botox may take care of some but not all the wrinkles you would like removed. In addition, we offer information about other wrinkle-removal procedures you can pursue with or without Botox. Ultimately, you and your physician will decide what's right for you.

How This Book Will Help You

Before you make that lunch date for your Botox injections, we invite you to read through this book. In it we discuss:

- CHAPTER 2: BOTOX: IS IT FOR YOU? In this chapter we discuss the questions you need to ask yourself honestly before you even begin to look for a practitioner. We also tell you about some medical situations that may not make you a candidate for Botox.

- CHAPTER 3: REALITY OF WRINKLES. As you look in the mirror you know those wrinkles are real enough. But how did they get there? They didn't just appear overnight. This chapter explains how wrinkles are born, how skin ages, and some things you can do to reduce the damaging effects of the sun.

- CHAPTER 4: THE BIRTH OF BOTOX AND HOW IT WORKS. The road to use of this toxin as a cosmetic enhancer has been one of scientific discovery and serendipity. In this chapter we talk about how the bacteria behind Botox were transformed from being a deadly poison to a welcome beauty product.

- CHAPTER 5: BEYOND BEAUTY: OTHER USES FOR BOTOX. For tens of thousands of people, Botox has been more than a wrinkle remover: it has significantly improved the physical and emotional quality of their lives. This chapter looks at the many medical uses of Botox, both those approved by the Food and Drug Administration and the off-label uses, some of which are currently being considered by the FDA. Who knows: someday you may be asking your doctor for Botox for something else besides wrinkles.

- CHAPTER 6: FINDING THE RIGHT DOCTOR. Who is best qualified to do Botox injections? This chapter discusses the qualifications you should look for when shop-

ping for a Botox physician, the questions you should ask
her or him, and the various organizations that can help
you by providing referrals as well as answering questions about the professionals or their qualifications. We
also discuss one of the potentially big drawbacks of
Botox: its cost.

- CHAPTER 7: WHAT TO EXPECT AT THE DOCTOR'S
  OFFICE. Let's say you've made the decision to have the
  injections. In this chapter we take you through a typical
  process: from your consultation, through the injections,
  and until the time you're back at work or at home; the
  next few hours and days as the Botox does its magic;
  and the subsequent weeks and months; and what to expect until you're ready for your next treatment.

- CHAPTER 8: SATISFACTION GUARANTEED? WHAT YOU
  NEED TO KNOW ABOUT SIDE EFFECTS AND COMPLICA-
  TIONS. Although Botox appears to offer the perfect way
  to eliminate certain types of wrinkles, there is also a
  downside. Admittedly, adverse effects seldom occur,
  but you should be aware of any negative reactions that
  may happen, why they can happen, and how to avoid
  them.

- CHAPTER 9: GOING BEYOND BOTOX: OTHER COS-
  METIC PROCEDURES. This chapter looks at other cosmetic procedures that are available for removing
  wrinkles. These options include chemical peels, the injection of filler materials (collagen, fat, AlloDerm,
  Cymetra, Gore-Tex, SoftForm), dermabrasion, and various laser procedures. These can be used along with, or
  instead of, Botox injections.

- CHAPTER 10: CARING FOR YOUR SKIN, FROM THE
INSIDE OUT AND THE OUTSIDE IN. Beauty really is
more than skin-deep, and that's because what you put
into your body has a way of showing on your skin. By
the same token, how well you treat your outer skin
layer matters when it comes to the development of lines
and wrinkles. This chapter discusses diet and nutritional supplements and how they can help your skin.
Then we talk about many of the ingredients you find in
skin care products, such as alpha hydroxy acids, collagen, copper, vitamin A, and vitamin E, and how they
may or may not help your skin or prevent wrinkles and
other signs of aging. Then we close with some advice on
choosing cleansers and moisturizers.

Maximizing Your Results

We want you to trust your face to the people most qualified to help you look your best. We also want you to be able
to look in the mirror each and every day and be satisfied with
what you see. You can be happy and successful and popular,
and whatever else you want to be, with or without wrinkles.
The choice is up to you. It's your face. Be good to it.

2

BOTOX: IS IT FOR YOU?

IF YOU ARE LIKE many men and women in America who have contemplated doing something about their lines and wrinkles, the sudden popularity of Botox and the reports from its many satisfied users intrigue you. You see where Botox *could* open up a new, exciting opportunity for you to eliminate those bothersome signs of aging. But before you make an appointment for Botox treatments, there are several questions you need to ask yourself, and first on the list is this: Is Botox right for you?

That is the question we will help you answer in this chapter. At first glance, the answer may seem simple: "Of course," you may be saying to yourself, "if Botox gets rid of my frown lines and crows'-feet, then it's right for me."

While beauty may be only skin-deep, the answer to the question "Is Botox right for me?" requires you to go a little deeper and to explore your motivations, expectations, and state of mind. We will help you look at those factors in this chapter and allow you to arrive at an answer to the question that is best for you.

BEAUTY AND YOUTH

Everywhere you look, you're reminded that beauty, youth, and attractiveness are highly desirable traits. You only need to watch television and movies or see the advertisements splashed in magazines and newspapers to know that youth is in, sexy sells, and wrinkles don't rock (except in a chair, that is).

But there's more to beauty than just looking good. We've already seen that if we believe we look good, we often perform better at work, in school, in social settings, and in relationships. It all comes down to self-esteem and self-confidence. And it comes down to what your idea of beauty is.

In some cultures, for example, long earlobes are found attractive. In others, a hint of facial hair above a woman's lip is considered sexy. Yet in the United States, women spend tens of thousands of dollars every year to have droopy earlobes fixed and to have their upper-lip hair removed with electrolysis or laser treatments. Likewise, in some societies, wrinkles are a sign of wisdom and demand a certain amount of respect.

America is in the grips of a youth-oriented culture. We may respect age and wisdom, but we want it to look younger than it really is. And with the growing number of advances in cosmetic techniques, we have more ways to look younger and to do it safely, quickly, and efficiently than ever before. Botox injections is one of those ways.

THE STIGMA IS GONE

Years ago, people who wanted to have a face-lift or an eyelid tuck created all kinds of elaborate excuses about why they were "disappearing" for a few weeks. Often they were afraid they would be labeled vain or conceited.

Today, the stigma of cosmetic surgery and other cosmetic procedures is fading fast. Worrying about what other people will think of them is becoming less of an issue.

"Everyone here basically gets cosmetic surgery if they can afford it, or if they need it, and it's no big deal," says Ronald Fragen, MD, of Fragen Cosmetic Surgery Center in Palm Springs, California, and a board member of the American Academy of Cosmetic Surgery. "There's no 'Am I being narcissistic?' by doing it. It's like a rite of passage: when someone feels they need it, they get it done."

It wasn't always that way. "I remember saying to myself, 'Just who does she think she is,' when my sister had a face-lift ten years ago," says Doreen, a sixty-seven-year-old manager of a floral shop. "I didn't think she needed it. My God, she's my baby sister! If she thought she needed a face-lift, what were people thinking about me!"

Doreen's sister made up an excuse, like many people years ago who made up stories about having to go away for a while, needing to go on a long business trip, or having had an accident. Doreen laughs when she remembers the excuse her sister gave everyone: "She said she had had an automobile accident and bumped her head, which was supposed to explain the bruising. I don't think anyone believed it."

The stigma hasn't vanished just in glamour cities like

Palm Springs and Hollywood. Dermatologists, plastic surgeons, cosmetic ophthalmologists, and other cosmetic surgeons all across the country are experiencing a boom in cosmetic procedures, especially those that can be accomplished quickly and easily in the office, with no downtime for the patient. And that's where Botox injections fit like a glove.

It's not just actors and actresses who are freely admitting to having cosmetic alterations. Secretaries, construction workers, nursery school teachers, truck drivers, and accountants are getting Botox and other cosmetic procedures, like collagen injections, during their lunch breaks. Friends, family, and coworkers are eagerly talking to other people about their experiences with Botox. The stigma appears to be quickly fading as cosmetic rejuvenation becomes more and more acceptable.

IS BOTOX FOR YOU?

Every woman and man who is considering Botox injections, and other cosmetic procedures that may also be necessary to achieve the look they desire, needs to do some soul-searching and homework before undergoing the procedure. Robert N. Butler, MD, gerontologist, president of the International Longevity Center in New York City, and Pulitzer Prize–winning author of the book *Why Survive? Being Old in America,* admits that "by and large, Botox injections are a relatively safe procedure. But my own philosophy in medicine has always been, if it's not broken, don't fix it. So although Botox seems to be relatively safe, I still think the person who seeks it should be fully informed of any of the dangers and should give some real thought to the question: Do I really want to have a smooth forehead?"

In order for you to decide if you need—or desire—to have a smooth forehead or to eliminate other troublesome wrinkles, you need to start with the basics and ask yourself: When I look in the mirror, what do I see—I mean *really* see?

- Do you see a person who is self-confident and poised, but who has a few wrinkles that she believes take away from her appearance and make her feel a little bit older on the outside than she feels inside?

- Do you see a person who is basically happy and full of energy, but who believes that getting rid of the lines between his eyes will make him look as young as he feels?

- Do you see a person who is depressed or who has just been hurt by a relationship gone bad and who believes that wiping out the crow's-feet and lines on her forehead will make her incredibly happy and ready to jump back into the dating scene?

- Do you see someone who believes that cosmetic procedures will make him or her perfect?

- Do you see a person who has lines and wrinkles but who feels happy and secure with herself, and who personally sees no reason why she should give in to the pressures society places on people to look young and beautiful?

The first two questions are about people who have a pretty realistic view of themselves. A "yes" to either of these questions indicates that you realize that getting Botox injections will enhance some part of your life, but it will not drastically change it. In other words, if for some reason the injections did not work, or if you were unable to continue to afford them, your life would not fall apart. You would adjust; life would go on. Perhaps you would consider another cosmetic procedure that would achieve your goal, but perhaps not.

If you see yourself answering "yes" to questions three or four, you need to stop and take a reality check. If you are depressed, anxious, experiencing feelings of despair or hopelessness, or generally feeling pessimistic about your life, your negative emotional state is coloring how you see yourself. The picture you see of yourself is distorted. You're in a state of mind that isn't best for making a big decision, such as whether or not you should have a cosmetic procedure.

Finally, if the last question describes you, then you're not a candidate for Botox. That's all right; Botox is not for everyone. Instead, pass this book along to a friend who may be contemplating getting the injections.

Making the Right Decision

"It sounded like a good idea at the time." Have you ever said this to yourself or to others about a decision you made? We've all done it, and chances are we'll do it again. But there's something gratifying about knowing that you made a decision after carefully weighing all your options and the risks and benefits, rather than just jumping in and then hoping you don't suffer any consequences.

You may have heard people who have had Botox injections, as well as doctors who give them, say that this procedure is "no big deal." And on one level that's true: you can have it done during your lunch break, there's no recovery time, side effects are virtually nil and transient, and wrinkles disappear within days.

Because we're talking about making changes to your face, albeit temporary ones, you should be certain that you want to make them for the right reasons, and that your expectations are realistic. To help you do that, try to be absolutely honest in answering the following questions. For the first few questions, you should be standing or sitting in a room that's well lit with natural light:

- Using a triple-magnification makeup mirror, look at your face. Where are the lines and wrinkles most noticeable? The forehead? Between your eyebrows? Around your eyes or mouth? Your cheeks? See the illustration on the next page to identify the lines on your face.

- Now put away that mirror and sit or stand in front of a regular mirror at a distance of about two feet. Look at your face again and ask yourself the same questions: How noticeable are these lines or wrinkles? Are they fine? Deep?

- Step back from the mirror to a distance of about five feet. Once again, look at your face. Are any of the lines and wrinkles you saw when you were looking closely at your face still visible?

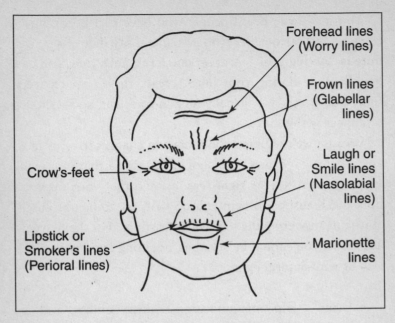

Forehead lines (Worry lines)

Frown lines (Glabellar lines)

Laugh or Smile lines (Nasolabial lines)

Crow's-feet

Lipstick or Smoker's lines (Perioral lines)

Marionette lines

Name That Wrinkle

Name That Wrinkle

From the top of your face down, bothersome facial wrinkles have the following names and locations. Notice that Botox is not the best choice for all types of wrinkles and lines. Other cosmetic options to eliminate wrinkles are discussed in chapter 9.

- Forehead lines: horizontal lines, often called worry lines. These lines form mainly because the underlying frontalis muscle, which stretches across the forehead, moves when you make facial expressions. When you lift your brow—sometimes referred to as the "aha" or surprised look—the muscle contracts, which causes the skin that is covering the muscle to pull, wrinkle, and then return to its original position when you relax the muscle. Now consider the countless number of times you've used these muscles. As you age, your skin begins to lose its elasticity, it suffers from sun damage, and the constant contracting and relaxing of the muscle results in forehead lines. These can be eliminated using Botox or filler injections such as collagen or fat.

- Frown lines: vertical lines, also known as glabellar lines, that appear between the eyebrows. These lines can make you appear serious, angry, or stressed even when you're not. It is for the removal of these lines that the Food and Drug Administration gave approval for Botox in April 2002. These lines are best removed with Botox. If you've frowned a lot over the years and the lines are very deeply etched, you may also need wrinkle fillers (e.g., collagen, fat) to eliminate these lines. Your doctor will discuss your options with you.

- Crow's-feet: lines that radiate from the outside corners of the eyes. They're also known as periorbital lines. If you have these lines, they're most likely the result of smiling and squinting. If you look in the mirror and smile or squint, notice how your muscles contract and cause your eyelids to nearly cover your eyes and how the muscles contract at the corners of your eyes where the lines appear. Crow's-feet are best eliminated with Botox, plus adjunctive treatment such as collagen, chemical peels, or laser resurfacing.

- Laugh lines: also known as smile lines or nasolabial lines, they are the two vertical lines that run from the outside corners of the nose down to the top of the outside of the upper lip. Even though they are called laugh lines, gravity and aging are also factors in their development. They can best be eliminated using wrinkle fillers (e.g., collagen, fat, AlloDerm, Cymetra, Gore-Tex, or SoftForm).

- Lipstick or smoker's lines: the tiny radiating lines that appear above the upper lip and below the lower one. It seems as though everyone has a different name for these annoying wrinkles, which are best removed using laser resurfacing, chemical peel, microdermabrasion, or wrinkle fillers—tissue augmentation (e.g., collagen injections, AlloDerm, fat)—in addition to Botox.

- Marionette lines: the often deep lines that run down from the outside corners of the mouth toward the chin. These lines develop from a combination of factors, including gravity (the cheeks tend to sag from the force of gravity) and thinning of the supporting tissue that comes with age. These wrinkles are best eliminated using wrinkle fillers or laser resurfacing. Another option is a face-lift, a complex surgical procedure that we do not discuss in this book.

Know Your Wrinkles. Although we haven't yet fully discussed all there is to know about Botox injections, you should know at this point that Botox injections work best on crow's-feet (wrinkles radiating from the outside corners of the eyes), worry lines (horizontal forehead lines), and frown lines (vertical lines, also called glabellar lines, that appear between the eyebrows). These are wrinkles that are typically caused by chronic contractions of the muscles under or adjacent to these areas of the face. Laughing, smiling, frowning, and squinting are some of the common facial expressions that can cause these lines. If you have lines and wrinkles on other parts of your face that concern you, you may need other types of cosmetic procedures to eliminate them. With that in mind, consider these questions:

- Which wrinkles and lines bother you the most? Are these lines and wrinkles the type that are best eliminated using Botox?

- If you choose to eliminate only the wrinkles that can be treated with Botox, will any of the remaining ones still leave you unsatisfied with your appearance? For example, if you want both your frown lines and marionette lines removed, you will likely need a different cosmetic procedure to have the marionette lines eliminated.

- If you'll still be bothered by the remaining lines and wrinkles, are you willing to have other cosmetic procedures done to correct them? Naturally, you will need to discuss all your options and prices with your doctor, but you should be aware that other procedures may be needed for you to get the look you desire. You also should know that while Botox injections don't involve any recovery time, some other cosmetic procedures do. (See chapter 9 for more information about other cosmetic procedures.)

Wrinkles and Your State of Mind. You also need to consider your state of mind before you decide to get Botox injections or any type of cosmetic procedure. It's possible that how you see your face is somewhat colored or distorted by your emotional state. Consider the following questions:

- Are you depressed? You may not have been formally diagnosed with depression, but if you meet the criteria for either of the following types of depression, major depression or mild depression (dysthymia) and you believe that having a cosmetic procedure will make them go away, you should talk to a mental health professional before you make a decision about undergoing cosmetic changes.

  For major depression, you must have one or both of these requirements: abnormal depressed mood most of the day, nearly every day, for at least two weeks; and/or abnormal loss of interest and pleasure most of the day, nearly every day, for at least two weeks. In addition, you must have at least five of the following present during the same two-week period:

  - Prolonged and chronic feelings of despair or sadness
  - Frequent irritability or anger
  - Difficulty concentrating or problems making decisions
  - Bouts of uncontrollable crying
  - Feelings of hopelessness and helplessness
  - Mood swings
  - Persistent brooding about the past and the way things were
  - Uncharacteristic loss of appetite or overeating
  - Sleep disturbances: wanting to sleep all the time or trouble sleeping

- Lack of interest in things that used to interest you, including hobbies, friends, and sex
- Lack of energy or motivation
- Abnormal thoughts of death or suicide

Mild depression is common, and is characterized by persistent feelings of sadness and low self-esteem, feeling depressed most of the day, more days than not, for at least two years, plus two or more of the following symptoms. During the past two years, you should never have been without two of these symptoms for more than two months:

- Poor appetite or overeating
- Wanting to sleep all the time or having trouble sleeping
- Fatigue
- Low self-esteem
- Poor concentration or difficulty making decisions
- Feelings of hopelessness

- Do you believe that eliminating your frown lines, crow's-feet, or other facial wrinkles will make any of the characteristics listed here go away?

- Do you believe that getting Botox injections will make you more popular, or that they will make your relationships, job, social life, or other aspects of your life perfect? Do you believe that the fact that you are aging is responsible for any unhappiness in your life?

- Is anyone else—a spouse, partner, family member, friend—pressuring you to have wrinkles removed? Or would undergoing Botox injections be something you would do for yourself alone?

Nancy's Story

Nancy, a forty-year-old administrative assistant, called her friend Carole and asked her for the name of her cosmetic surgeon. Six months prior, Carole had had Botox injections to remove her frown lines and crow's-feet, and a chemical peel to eliminate some other fine facial wrinkles. As a high school principal, Carole, age forty-six, was always in the public eye, meeting with school administrators, parents, and school board members. But she felt that looking a little younger would help her relationships with her students rather than with her peers.

"Being able to relate to my students is very important to me," she says. "I didn't have these procedures done to look like my students. I just wanted to close the generation gap a little so the students may be more willing to keep the communication lines with me open."

But when Carole got the call from Nancy, she questioned her friend's motives for wanting cosmetic surgery. "I knew Nancy was going through some rough times," says Carole. "She's a single mom, and her teenage daughter had been giving her some problems. And she'd been pretty depressed for several years, ever since her husband left her."

Nancy is also the type that reads all the self-help books, believing they will help her simply by osmosis. "I got the impression from her call that she thought having her face redone would completely change her life for the better," says Carole.

Fortunately, Carole has an understanding cosmetic surgeon who, after talking with Nancy, was able to convince her that she had unrealistic expectations about what changing her looks would do for her life. With some coaxing from Carole and the doctor, Nancy enrolled in a depression study at a local medical facility and began taking an antidepressant. Eight months later, she went back to the cosmetic surgeon and asked for Botox "just to get rid of the frown lines. I don't feel sad anymore, and so I don't want to look like I'm frowning all the time."

Do It for You

When you're standing in front of the mirror evaluating what you see, is there someone standing over your shoulder telling you what to see? Harold had such a "someone."

"My wife means well," says Harold, a fifty-six-year-old electrical engineer. "She gets Botox treatments, and they make her look great. Of course, I thought she looked great before the treatments, but she wanted to have them. I certainly had no objection; she should be able to do what makes her feel good."

But Harold wants to do what makes him feel good as well, and, he says, getting Botox injections isn't on his list. He's had some trouble convincing his wife that he's happy with his face the way it is.

The only person you need to please when you're thinking about getting Botox injections or other cosmetic procedures is you: not your spouse, boyfriend, girlfriend, mother, sister, or best friend. Whenever you do something just to please someone else, chances are you'll resent the other person for "making" you do it. Yet you're the one who will have to live with the decision. Of course, in the case of Botox injections, the effects fade after three to six months, and you'll need to get another treatment if you want to keep the wrinkle-free look. That gives you the luxury of choosing another cosmetic option, getting another treatment, or putting your foot down with your "persuasive" partner and saying it's not for you.

If you decide to do Botox, do it for you.

Botox: Yes . . . and No

For one young woman, Botox turned out to be exactly what she wanted . . . and exactly what she didn't want, both at the same time. Madelaine, a thirty-six-year-old social worker, went to her dermatologist looking for two things: a way to eliminate the horizontal wrinkles in her forehead and a way to stop a small muscle spasm that affected one side of her face. The spasm was intermittent; it usually occurred several times a day but occasionally more often, and it had been happening for about two years.

Madelaine had read in a magazine how Botox temporarily relaxed muscles and how it was used for various conditions that involved involuntary muscle movements. When she sat down with her dermatologist to discuss her options, he suggested Botox for her forehead wrinkles, because they were the result of her tendency to scrunch her forehead, but discouraged it for the muscle spasm. His concern, he told her, was that injecting the toxin into the muscle would relax or weaken it, which could cause her face to droop on the treated side and appear as if she had had a stroke.

Madelaine believed the twitch was distracting to her clients, and she was willing to try Botox, even though she fully understood that it might not work. After her doctor explained the risks and said that if the face droop did occur, it would dissipate within several months, she opted to try the injection.

As predicted, Madelaine's face drooped on the one side, and after three months it returned to normal. She continues to get her Botox treatments for her forehead lines, but she has also learned to live with her facial twitch. "I think it probably bothered me more than it does anyone else," she says. "Actually, having the droopy face bothered me a lot more than the twitch ever did. Now, I'm so happy that I got rid of my frown lines that having the twitch isn't such a big deal anymore."

Not Everyone Is a Candidate

Although getting Botox injections is a safe procedure, it should not be undertaken if certain health and medical conditions exist. You should not take Botox if you are pregnant or breast-feeding, or if you are taking quinine, penicillamine, or the aminoglycoside antibiotics tobramycin, vancomycin, or gentamicin. Fortunately, these are usually temporary situations. You won't be pregnant or breast-feeding forever; you may be taking aminoglycosides for only a few weeks. Once your situation changes, it will probably be safe for you to get the injections.

If, however, you have muscle-weakening conditions such as multiple sclerosis, myasthenia gravis, polymyositis, Bell's palsy, or Lou Gehrig's disease, you are not a candidate for Botox. If you have a skin infection or a type of dermatitis (an inflammatory skin condition such as contact dermatitis or poison ivy) in the area you want treated, you should wait until the condition has cleared before getting the injections.

All of these health and medical questions will be brought up during your interview or consultation, but it's a good idea to know about them now so you can consider them in your decision-making process.

THE PRICE OF BEAUTY

When deciding if Botox is right for you, the cost of treatments needs to be a consideration as well. Botox injections, when given for cosmetic reasons, are not covered by insurance. (There are medical uses for Botox, some of which are usually covered by insurance. These are discussed in chapter 5.) Therefore, you must consider whether your desire to get Botox matches your ability to pay. Each site that is treated (e.g., for frown lines, crow's-feet, or forehead lines) can cost about $200 to $600 or even more, depending on the amount of Botox you need (as measured in units). Some people need more of the drug than others. To maintain the look you want, you'll need two to three treatments per year, typically one every four to six months. Naturally, you can decide to stop at any time, and there will be no side effects. However, if you plan to continue getting the injections, you will need to make sure you can afford the additional impact on your budget.

For Pamela, a forty-one-year-old divorced mother of two, the ability to pay for her Botox treatments was a stretch, but she was willing to make the adjustments to her lifestyle to get what she wanted. "When I was trying to decide whether I could afford to get Botox injections, I promised myself that I'd give up a few things if I had to, as long as I never took anything away from what my children needed." For Pamela, that meant brown-bagging her lunch instead of eating out, cutting down on take-out dinners, and cooking at home instead.

"It works out that my kids and I eat better now, and I save a lot of money, money I put away to pay for my injections," she says. "And once I stopped eating out, I found that I actually saved more than I needed for the Botox. So I'm coming out ahead all around!"

Pamela realizes that a day may come when other expenditures prevent her from continuing the injections. "That's okay with me," she says. "I'm enjoying the look they give me while I can."

* * *

The bottom line is, if your expectation is that Botox injections or other cosmetic procedures will dramatically improve your life, that your life will be perfect once your wrinkles are gone, or that other people will love or appreciate you more once your wrinkles disappear, then you're probably not a candidate for Botox injections or any cosmetic procedure at this time. Or, as one doctor says, if you have wrinkles all over and you're only going to do something about one or two, why bother?

None of this means you never will or never should have Botox. But before you take the step and get the injections, you should be fully realistic about the outcome, be comfortable with your decision, and know that you're doing it for no one but yourself.

You may also be an individual who wants the look Botox can provide but who is not comfortable having a drug injected into her forehead. And that's okay. There are several other cosmetic options you can pursue. You should talk to a qualified professional (see chapter 6) who can explain all the options to you and help you choose an alternative (read about some of them in chapter 9) that will give you the look you desire.

QUESTIONS AND ANSWERS

Several of my friends are getting Botox injections and they are pressuring me to get them too. I have some wrinkles around my eyes and on my forehead, but they don't bother me very much. What should I do?

You said it yourself—"pressuring." You should not undergo Botox or any other cosmetic procedure to please anyone but yourself. Your friends may mean well, but you are

the one who has to live with the decision and the consequences of your decision (and the cost). If you do not feel you
need Botox, then do not get it. Plus, if you did get the injections, you might resent that your friends pressured you into
it, and you might feel angry at yourself for allowing them to
pressure you. It's your face; you should do what feels best for
you. Besides, you can tell them that with the money you're
saving by not having the injections, you're going to treat
yourself to something special.

*I'd like to get Botox for my frown lines, but the cost is a fac-
tor. I may be able to afford it if insurance pays part of each
treatment. Does insurance cover Botox injections?*

Cost is definitely an issue you should consider when deciding if you are a candidate for Botox, because in order to
keep the wrinkle-free look, you must keep going back for
treatments about every four to six months. No, insurance
does not cover cosmetic procedures. You must pay for them
out of your own pocket. Costs vary from one doctor to the
next and include a product plus an administration fee.

*I told my dermatologist that I wanted to get Botox injections
for my crow's-feet, but she said because I am six-months
pregnant, she wants me to wait until I have my baby. Why do
I need to wait? Could Botox be harmful to my baby?*

Your dermatologist is wise to advise you this way. Although indications are that the toxin stays in the area into
which it is injected and thus should not be transmitted to a
fetus, a cautious approach is best. No studies have been done
to determine whether Botox injections have any effect on a
fetus, or whether Botox can be transmitted in breast milk.

My twenty-five-year high school reunion is coming up in a few months, and I'm considering Botox injections for my frown lines and crow's-feet. My husband thinks it's a waste of money to get injections for just one time. Is there any harm in getting just one treatment?

Some celebrities get the injections for special events, so why should you be any different? You don't seem to have any unrealistic expectations about Botox—you merely want to look your best for a big occasion. You realize, of course, that you may like the results so much that you'll want to go back again and again. That's probably the biggest risk you're taking.

There's a man who goes to my health club whose attention I've been trying to get for months, but he doesn't seem to be very interested. I've noticed that he likes younger women (he's forty-three, I'm forty-four). I want to get Botox injections for my forehead, crow's-feet, and lines around my mouth so I'll look younger. My sister says I'm crazy. What do you think?

We don't agree with your sister, but we do think you should reconsider why you want to get the injections. If your only reason for getting the injections is to impress a man who hasn't paid much attention to you up to this point, you should ask yourself: Do I want someone who is only interested in how young I look? Or do I want someone who will truly appreciate me for all I am? Botox injections, and other cosmetic procedures, are an enhancement of the person you already are inside.

What if you get the injections and he still doesn't pay any attention to you? Will you be devastated? What if he has another girlfriend by the time your treatments take effect? We suggest you reconsider your decision.

3

REALITY OF WRINKLES

THE UNFORTUNATE TRUTH is that exposure to the sun is the major cause of wrinkles. More specifically, photo damage from the sun is the main factor in causing wrinkles, and about 80 percent of the sun damage has been done to our skin by the time we are eighteen years of age.

"If I only knew then what I know now," laments Claudia, a forty-eight-year-old Realtor living in Virginia. "My mother didn't think about sunscreen when I was a kid, and so I didn't think much about it when I got older. All I cared about was getting a tan and looking good." She shakes her head as she looks in the mirror. "Well, I have the tan, but it's not looking so good right now, not with all the wrinkles and lines on my face. I'm beginning to look like a piece of crinkled leather."

All those summer days Claudia spent "working" on her tan paid her back when she reached her thirties and natural aging began to catch up with the sun damage.

OF AGING SKIN AND WRINKLES

Soft as a baby's bottom. Ah, if we could only keep that soft, fresh, wrinkle-free skin forever. But this wonderful body covering has many functions to perform, and one of them is to protect what lies beneath it. That means our skin is constantly exposed to the environment and all it has to throw our way—including ultraviolet rays from the sun, water, air pollutants, and chemicals and other irritants found in soaps, lotions, cleaning products, and cosmetics.

Our skin not only helps keep us cool by producing sweat, it also protects us from the cold, wards off invading disease-causing organisms, and produces vitamin D from the sun. It reflects our emotions—you can be white with fear, flushed with embarrassment, red with rage, or covered with goosebumps when you get cold—and it can tingle with pleasure when touched. And like every other organ (skin is the body's largest organ), it is affected by the passage of time.

The groundwork for wrinkles actually begins during childhood, even though you likely won't see the damaging results of sun exposure for several decades. So while you're feeling good about getting a great tan, the sun has other plans for your skin.

To help understand how sun damage results in wrinkles and other signs of aging, it helps to know the skin you're in. Human skin is actually a complex structure, composed of two main layers: the epidermis and the dermis. Each of these layers is composed of several sublayers and components, all of which play a role in how your skin ages and wrinkles. Let's take a close look at your skin.

What You See: Epidermis

The top layer of skin is called the epidermis, which is about as thick as one or two pages in a book. Its main function is to produce keratin, a protein that protects us against injury and helps skin to retain its moisture. The epidermis is protected by the stratum corneum, a superficial layer of dead cells that is constantly being shed from the skin's surface as new cells are produced below and move up to the surface. This sublayer is what you typically see as your skin.

This process of cell replacement takes about 28 days when we're in our twenties or thirties. That's good news, because who wants all those dead cells hanging around? But as we age, that 28-day period gradually gets longer and longer. As

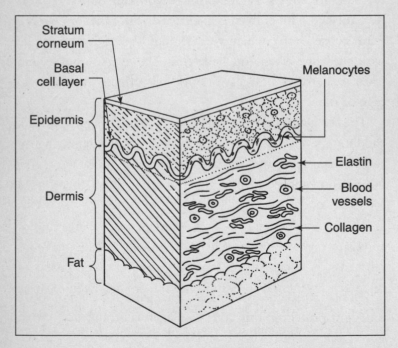

Anatomy of the Skin

we approach sixty and seventy, it can take six to eight weeks for the cells to be shed. Perhaps now you can appreciate why older skin doesn't have the glow or fresh look that younger skin has.

At the bottom of the epidermis layer are basal cells, which are the new cells that migrate to the stratum corneum and are eventually shed. Pigment cells called melanocytes are also found in the epidermis. These cells contain the pigment melanin, which helps protect the skin against the harmful ultraviolet (UV) rays. The more melanin you have, the more protection you have. That's why people who have naturally darker skin, such as African-Americans, Native Americans, and people of Mediterranean descent, have more protection against the damaging effects of UV rays and typically have fewer wrinkles.

In fact, many people who have black skin have a built-in sun-protection factor (SPF) of 13, depending on the darkness of their skin. Even with this inherent protection, they, too, should wear sunscreen, because they are prone to developing dark blotches from sun exposure.

The Dermis: Birthplace of Wrinkles

The dermis is an area rich in components that give skin its support and structure. When these components are damaged, either by natural aging processes or by outside factors such as ultraviolet rays, wrinkles are formed. That's why the dermis is the birthplace of wrinkles.

One of those components is collagen, which is the most abundant protein in this layer. Collagen is arranged in interwoven strands and provides the skin with strength and structure. Elastin fibers, another critical component found in the dermis, are true to their name: they provide elasticity, or the ability to rebound from pressure to or stretching of the skin.

Floating among the collagen and elastin strands are substances that help enhance your skin's texture and maintain an adequate water level to keep your tissues hydrated. These components include ceramides, hyaluronic acids, glycerin, and polysaccharides, among others. These components also decrease in number as we age. Yet one more critical element in the dermis is the network of blood vessels, which nourish the skin.

Although wrinkles appear on your epidermis, they are nurtured in the dermis and are thus the tip of the iceberg, so to speak. As we age, the number of collagen and elastin fibers decreases and those that remain are stretched or damaged. The majority of the damage comes from exposure to the sun, but other factors also play a role, including heredity and hormone fluctuations (also see "Other Factors That Age the Skin," further on in this chapter, for other wrinkle makers).

But again, the biggest culprit is the sun. And you *can* do something about your exposure to the sun, as you'll learn later in this chapter.

Friendly Fat

Although we often tend to bad-mouth fat, there are times and situations in our lives when fat is very desirable. And skin health is one of them. It's a sad fact that as we age, the number of fat cells in the dermis declines. This is one reason why older skin looks thinner and more transparent than younger skin. People who are overweight also have thinner skin as they age, but they tend to have fewer wrinkles for another reason: the fat responsible for their weight lies in another layer below the dermis—the subcutis (sub = below; cutis = skin) fat layer. This layer is not considered to be part of the skin, but we mention it because it helps keep your skin "plumped out" and less prone to wrinkling. Therefore, the less fat you have, the more susceptible you can be to wrinkling.

How Sun Exposure Damages the Skin

The damage to your skin begins in the form of ultraviolet (UV) rays that radiate from the sun in three forms: UVA, UVB, and UVC. You don't have to worry about the UVC rays, because most of them are filtered out by the earth's ozone layer high in the atmosphere.

But beware of UVA and UVB rays, the bad boys when it comes to wrinkles and aging skin, and the rays you want to block with sunscreen (see below). Ultraviolet rays penetrate the skin and trigger free radical production as a result of cellular damage. These free radicals then cause further cell damage. Free radicals are molecules that are unstable because they are missing an electron. In order to make themselves stable, they seek out other molecules and steal electrons from them, which is how more free radicals are created.

The more you expose your skin to ultraviolet rays, the more free radicals are created. When free radicals are created, the process causes cell damage, including damage to collagen, elastin, and other components of the skin. This damage results in wrinkles, loss of elasticity, brown spots, and other signs of aging skin. While youthful, healthy skin has the ability to clear itself of free radicals and the damage they can cause, skin that is exposed to UV light cannot.

Ultraviolet rays also cause your skin to age in another way, as they stimulate an enzyme that is responsible for breaking down the fat in your skin cells. Although breaking down fat may sound like a good thing, especially if you're trying to lose a few pounds, in this case the results are not so good. As the fat breaks down, a substance called arachidonic acid is produced, which ultimately causes the skin to age faster.

You're not out of danger yet. Ultraviolet light can also trigger special molecules in your skin cells to produce enzymes that digest collagen, a protein that gives your skin its flexibility and strength. So as the years go by and the UV rays keep penetrating your skin, these enzymes keep destroying your collagen, leaving you with less and less.

The result of all this sun exposure?

- Thinner skin
- Less elastic skin
- Sagging skin
- Skin cancer and precancer
- Age spots (brown/liver spots)
- Wrinkles

"But," you insist, "I was never a sun-worshipper. I didn't lay on the beach. I never got sunburn." Despite popular opinion, you don't need to get a sunburn to have sun damage and aging skin. The fact is, skin that is exposed, unprotected, to ultraviolet rays will age. Even driving a car or sitting by a window exposes you to the sun's rays, because although UVB rays are blocked by the glass, UVA rays are not.

Assessing Sun Damage: A Test

If you're still not convinced that the sun is responsible for the majority of lines, wrinkles, and aging on your face, conduct this small experiment. This test works best if you're older than forty and not more than 20 pounds over your ideal weight (that's because fat helps keep wrinkles at bay). However, if you're younger than forty and you have wrinkles on your face, you should take this test, too.

Look carefully at the skin on your face and note its texture, the presence of fine lines and wrinkles, and any other characteristics that bother you. Then take a look at the skin on your buttocks. (Use that full-length mirror hiding behind your bedroom door.) If you are like most people, you haven't made a practice of exposing your bare buttocks to the sun, so you should see a dramatic difference between the skin on your face and that on your derriere. True, your buttocks may be sagging a bit, but what we're interested in here is the fact that your derriere does not have wrinkles or fine lines; it is probably smooth and even in color and tone. But your face, because it has been exposed to the sun for decades, and because of other factors we talk about below, shows the signs of that exposure. And the farther away from forty you are, the more pronounced this difference will likely be.

Other Factors That Age the Skin

Exposure to the sun isn't the only thing that causes your skin to age. Let's say you've been careful about how much time you spend in the sun. You wear sunscreen. You follow the guidelines we outline in the following box (see "Protecting Your Skin"). And yet there they are, staring back at you in the mirror: the furrowed brow, the laugh lines (but you're not laughing), and the crow's-feet. You're probably wondering why you still have wrinkles when you were so careful.

That's because there are other factors that contribute to

wrinkles and aging skin. We've already talked a great deal about exposure to the sun, which is responsible for about 80 percent of the age-related changes that occur to your face. But the remaining 20 percent can play a significant role in the formation of fine lines and wrinkles. Here are some of those factors:

- Smoking. It seems there is an endless list of reasons not to smoke, and here are yet some more. Cigarette smoking robs the body of vitamin C, which is a critical component in the production of collagen. Smoking also reduces the blood supply to the skin, which means less oxygen to the cells, resulting in coarser, thicker facial skin that wrinkles more easily. And when you think about the physical movement involved in smoking—the pursing of the lips as you inhale—you can see how and why wrinkles form around the mouth.

- Environmental factors, such as air pollutants and secondhand smoke. These factors promote the production and activity of free radicals, which accelerate the aging process and promote fine lines and wrinkles.

- Irritating soaps, cleansers, and skin lotions. You want to use products that are kind to your face. See chapter 10 for a discussion on the best soaps and moisturizers to promote healthy skin.

- A poor diet. The Standard American Diet, or SAD, is really just that, because it is typically deficient in fiber and nutrients that help promote healthy skin, such as vitamins A, C, and E. We discuss diet and nutrition and their role in healthy skin in more detail in chapter 10.

- Sleep. Some dermatologists can tell their patients exactly which side or part of their face they sleep on by looking at the wrinkles on their face. Think about how you sleep and then look at the wrinkles on your face. Could some of them be caused or made worse by the way you sleep on your pillow? You can try sleeping on your back, which eliminates any pressure on your face, or using a soft pillow that has a satin pillowcase to minimize the effect on your skin. Another sleep concern is getting enough. If you are often sleep deprived, as many Americans are, your muscles become fatigued, including those in your face, and your skin begins to sag, contributing to the formation of wrinkles, especially in the lower half of your face.

- Stress. When you're tense, stressed-out, or angry, you tighten your muscles, not just those in your neck and shoulders, but also those in your face. A tense, stressed face promotes wrinkles, especially around the eyes, on the bridge of the nose, and along the forehead. These wrinkles are the type that can be eliminated with Botox, because they are caused by contractions of the muscles in the face. Botox relaxes and paralyzes those muscles, causing the wrinkles to soften and fade away. Chronic stress can also deprive your skin of nutrients and oxygen.

- Alcohol consumption. We're not saying you shouldn't enjoy an occasional drink, but think before you drink. Alcohol increases the amount of fluid leakage from the tiny blood vessels called capillaries. This causes more fluids to be transported from the bloodstream into your soft tissues. If you drink alcohol within one to two hours of going to sleep, the combination of lying down and the movement of fluids into the soft tissues can cause the skin to stretch and promote wrinkle formation.

Protecting Your Skin

It's never too late to protect your skin from harmful ultraviolet rays. Follow these guidelines to help prevent the promotion of wrinkling and signs of aging:

- **Invest in sunscreen.** It's your number-one protection against harmful ultraviolet rays. Use a sunscreen that provides protection against both UVA and UVB rays: it should state this on the label. Also, look for a product that provides a sun-protection factor (SPF) of at least 15; higher numbers are believed to provide even more protection. The Food and Drug Administration recommends using a sunscreen with an SPF up to 30; anything higher doesn't provide much additional protection.

- **Be generous.** Sunscreen should be applied liberally to provide maximum protection. "Liberally" means one ounce applied about 30 minutes before you go outside. And once is not enough: you need to keep reapplying the same amount every few hours, especially if you are sweating or going into the water.

- **Make it year-round.** Sunscreen should be applied every day of the year, in the summer, winter, spring, and fall, even when it's cloudy or hazy. Ultraviolet rays are always around, even on a cloudy day. Remember, too, that clouds, water, snow, concrete, and white sand reflect ultraviolet rays and increase your exposure to them.

- **Read the label.** When shopping for sunscreen, read the ingredient label. Any ingredient that ends in "-salicylate" or "-cinnamate" will protect you from UVB rays but not UVAs. The same goes for the ingredients PABA (para-aminobenzoic acid) and Padimate-O (octyl dimethyl para). The ingredient avobenzone (Parsol 1789) blocks only UVA rays. You want a product that blocks both types of rays, so look for those that contain oxybenzone, titanium dioxide, or zinc oxide.

- **Test your sunscreen.** Some people's skin is sensitive to certain ingredients in sunscreen. Before you apply a new sunscreen all over your face, apply a small amount to your inner arm. If you don't have a reaction (itching, redness) within an hour or so, it's probably safe. If you are sensitive to the product, you may want to find a chemical-free sunscreen.

- **Cover up.** Wear a hat with a 6- to 12-inch brim to shade your face, long sleeves, pants, a long skirt, or a long wrap to cover your arms and legs.

- **Stay out of beds.** Tanning beds, that is. Many people erroneously believe that tanning salons are safer than natural sunlight when it comes to burning or wrinkling. Tanning beds put out damaging ultraviolet rays that are guaranteed to age your skin. Avoid them.

- **Avoid midday sun.** The sun is typically most harmful to your skin between the hours of 10 AM and 3 PM. If you are outside during those hours, make sure you're wearing sunscreen and protective clothing.

- **Wear sunscreen with makeup.** If you wear makeup, you can purchase cosmetics that contain sunscreen, or apply your sunscreen under your makeup. Many liquid foundations contain sunscreen.

QUESTIONS AND ANSWERS

I still think a tan looks great, but I'm worried about the damage it does to my skin. How safe are the self-tanning products?

Self-tanning products, sometimes referred to as sunless tanners, bronzers, or tanning extenders, allow you to get a tanned look without spending time in the sun. They can do this because they contain a color additive that interacts with the amino acids in the surface of your skin. The only color additive that has been approved by the Food and Drug Administration for this purpose is DHA (dihydroxyacetone).

These products appear to be safe, but their appeal varies and depends on what you expect from the product. The chemicals in the various products can react differently on different areas of your body and cause an uneven tan. Some streak or run when your skin gets wet, although great advances have been made in many of the most popular products. Nearly all of them will stain your clothing, however, so you need to be careful when handling them.

You should not assume that a self-tanning or bronzer product will protect you against the sun's ultraviolet rays. Some of these products contain sunscreen ingredients and are labeled with SPF numbers; others are not. Always read the label carefully, especially if you plan to be out in the sun while wearing any of these products.

Is dry skin a cause of wrinkles?

It's a misconception that dry skin causes wrinkles. Dry skin appears to be more wrinkled than oily skin, which is why when you apply moisturizer to dry skin, the appearance of fine lines and wrinkles is reduced. In fact the phrase "reduces the appearance of fine lines and wrinkles" is one that manufacturers of moisturizers often use to sell their products. No moisturizer will *eliminate* wrinkles because it does nothing to fill them in or plump them out from under the skin.

What is SPF and what do the numbers mean?

SPF stands for sun-protection factor, and it's a measure of a sunscreen's ability to prevent your skin from getting sunburned for a specified period of time. The numbers tell you how much longer you can be exposed to the sun's rays without getting burned if you are wearing the product as opposed to not wearing any type of sunscreen at all.

For example, if your skin, unprotected by sunscreen, usually gets sunburned in 10 minutes and you apply a sunscreen with an SPF of 15, you can stay in the sun 15 times longer (or 2 hours and 30 minutes—150 minutes) before you will begin to burn. This 150-minute grace period depends, of course, on you applying an adequate amount of sunscreen and reapplying it as needed, which should be about every two hours and more often if you go into the pool or perspire a lot.

How long can I keep sunscreens? Do they have an expiration date?

If you have sunscreen and are using it properly, you shouldn't have to worry about the expiration date, because you'll be applying it every day. But sunscreens do have an expiration date, and you should note it when you make your purchase, especially if the product is on sale, as the expiration date may be close. Sunscreens typically have a shelf life of about one year. You can tell if your sunscreen is old and ineffective if it feels gritty, which means the chemicals have separated from the solution. That means it's time to throw the product away and get a new one. As a rule of thumb, if there's no expiration date, replace your sunscreen in one year.

How safe are tanning beds and sunlamps? My sister says they don't harm your skin nearly as much as the sun does.

Tanning beds and sunlamps are less likely to cause a sunburn, so many people think they're safer than lying in the sun. However, that's because tanning beds and sunlamps emit ultraviolet A rather than ultraviolet B rays. Ultraviolet B rays cause sunburn; ultraviolet A radiation is very damaging to the dermis, and specifically to collagen and elastin, and has been associated with skin aging and cancer. Thus tanning beds and sunlamps are breeding grounds for wrinkled, dry, leathery skin. Ultraviolet A rays also may contribute to the development of melanoma, a type of skin cancer. The Food and Drug Administration (FDA) and the Centers for Disease Control and Prevention (CDC) encourage people not to use these products.

Why do I need to wear sunscreen when it's cloudy?

According to the American Academy of Family Physicians, 60 to 80 percent of ultraviolet rays can get through the clouds and impact your skin. If the cloud cover is especially heavy, that percentage is closer to zero. Remember, too, that UV rays can also reach at least one foot below the water, so swimmers beware.

How does smoking cause wrinkles?

If you watch people who smoke, you can see how their lips are pursed when they inhale. This movement creates grooves in the skin around the mouth. Now multiply that movement by perhaps hundreds of times a day, then by the week, month, and year. The result: lots of small wrinkles radiating from the lips. According to one study, heavy smokers are nearly five times more likely to have wrinkled facial skin than nonsmokers.

Smoking also reduces the amount of oxygen that circulates in the bloodstream. Therefore the skin, which is rich in blood vessels, is deprived of adequate amounts oxygen and the nutrients carried in the bloodstream. The reduction in oxygen in the blood is the main reason doctors tell their patients to stop smoking several weeks before and after many cosmetic procedures (or any surgery for that matter), because the decline in oxygen hinders the healing process.

4

THE BIRTH OF BOTOX AND HOW IT WORKS

MANY PEOPLE HAVE WONDERED: Can a potentially lethal drug be used safely? The answer is clearly and substantively "yes."

Sandra had wondered the same thing before she decided six months ago to get her first Botox treatment. "I decided to get Botox because I was re-entering the job market at thirty-eight after having two children, and I knew competition was stiff," she says. Sandra, who landed a job as an acquisitions editor for a major book publisher, says she believes eliminating the prominent wrinkles on her forehead and around her eyes helped her feel more confident during her interviews. And, she says, she definitely looks younger.

But when she was trying to decide if Botox was right for her, she had some concerns about allowing a "poison" to be injected into her face. "I know everyone was saying it was safe," she says, "and I didn't have any reason not to believe the reports. But I've always been a curious person, and I wanted to know how a substance that can kill you can safely take away wrinkles. How did anyone come to that conclusion?"

As often happens in the realm of medicine, the discovery that this deadly toxin had health benefits was a case of science with a dose of serendipity.

THE BIRTH OF BOTOX

Around 1817, a German doctor and poet named Justinus Kerner published the first full description of the symptoms of an illness that was associated with eating tainted food. The illness, called botulism ("botulism" comes from the Latin "botulus," meaning "sausage"), was so named because it affected people who ate spoiled sausage. In those days, the symptoms of double vision, slurred speech, drooping eyelids, and muscle weakness soon progressed to muscle paralysis throughout the body, and death was often the result of paralysis of the muscles necessary for breathing.

Then in 1897, a microbiologist named Emile-Pierre van Ermengen isolated the bacterium *Clostridium botulinum*, which causes botulism. He extracted the organism both from the tissues of people who had died of the illness in Belgium, and from the offending food, which was raw, salted pork.

This bacterium *(C. botulinum)* produces eight different toxins, labeled A through G (with C1 and C2), and seven of them are capable of causing paralysis. The A serotype is the most potent, and that is the one being used most often today for both medical and cosmetic reasons, and the one found (highly diluted) in the drug sold under the trade name Botox.

Van Ermengen wasn't able to identify the exact toxin produced by *C. botulinum* that caused the people to die. That honor fell to Edward J. Schantz in 1946, when he isolated and purified the paralyzing botulinum toxin A. Years later, Schantz's work caught the attention of Alan B. Scott, MD, of the Smith-Kettlewell Eye Research Foundation, one of the pioneers of the medical uses of botulinum. Dr. Scott had been looking for a nonsurgical way to treat crossed eyes, or strabismus, by weakening the eye muscles responsible for the disorder.

When Scott started collaborating with Schantz, he found what he had been looking for: when minute amounts of botulinum toxin A were injected into the eye muscles of monkeys who had crossed eyes, their symptoms were relieved. From monkeys he moved on to human studies, and his success with strabismus in humans led him to try Botox in another eye disorder, blepharospasm, which involves involuntary spasms of the eye. (Both eye disorders are described below.) Again, he injected the botulinum toxin into the muscles around the eye, and the improvement was impressive.

Those success stories and others prompted investigators to complete and submit all the required research and trial data to the Food and Drug Administration (FDA) for approval of the drug. In 1989, the FDA approved Botox for the treatment of strabismus and blepharospasm. In the meantime, other researchers recognized that botulinum toxin A was useful in the treatment of other types of neuromuscular spasm disorders, known collectively as dystonias, and the studies began.

A cosmetic use for Botox had yet to be uncovered. Soon, however, science and serendipity came together.

THE ROAD FROM SPASMS TO WRINKLES

While doctors were injecting Botox into the eye and facial muscles of people who had various eye disorders involving involuntary muscle activity, they noticed a side benefit: facial wrinkles in the area of the injections were disappearing. These included frown lines (vertical lines that appear between the eyebrows directly above the nose), crow's-feet (lines that radiate from the outside corners of the eyes), and forehead lines (horizontal lines in the forehead).

Two physicians in particular—the wife-and-husband team of ophthalmologist Jean Carruthers and dermatologist J. Alastair Carruthers—noted that Dr. Scott's blepharospasm patients were enjoying the benefit of disappearing wrinkles after their Botox injections. Indeed, Dr. Scott indicated that he had used the toxin for cosmetic purposes during the 1980s. The Drs. Carruthers wrote about their findings in 1992, and their work was followed up by other investigators as well, among them Dr. Mitchell Brin and his group at Columbia University College of Physicians and Surgeons in New York.

Because Botox already had FDA approval for several conditions, doctors were legally and ethically allowed to use it for other medical disorders, the earlier noted practice called "off-label" use. As more and more doctors noted this beneficial side effect, they told their colleagues at meetings and conferences. As studies corroborated clinical experience, the Botox story spread like wildfire, mostly among dermatologists.

Few things spread faster than information about a beauty enhancer that really works. Thus, satisfied patients were soon on the phone telling all their friends about the wonderful new, quick way to eliminate wrinkles. One thing rapidly became clear: considering society's love affair with looking young and the anti-aging revolution, anything that could effectively and safely make wrinkles disappear would be a huge hit.

HOW BOTOX WORKS

"I know Botox isn't some kind of magic potion," says Stephanie, a fifty-eight-year-old librarian who has been getting Botox injections for more than two years. "When I first went for a consultation with my doctor, he explained how Botox works. But it's still magic to me."

Botox is a drug that contains botulinum toxin type A, a protein that is produced by the bacterium, *Clostridium botulinum*. The drug is classified as a neurotoxin, which means it has the ability to attack certain nerve cells and inhibit the transmission of nerve impulses.

The protein is purified, freeze-dried, and mixed with human serum albumin (a protein obtained from healthy blood donors and a common vehicle for injectable medications) and sodium chloride (salt, another common vehicle). It is packaged in 100-unit vials and delivered to doctors, who then mix it with a sterile salt solution when they are ready to use it as an injectable.

When the drug is injected into the muscle, it attaches itself to the nerve endings in the treated area and interferes with the release of a chemical called acetylcholine. Preventing the release of acetylcholine causes neurotransmitter binding sites to bundle up and atrophy (decrease in size) and stop the nerve signals from triggering the muscle contractions that are contributing to the wrinkles—or, when the drug is used for medical purposes, the muscle spasms. When the muscles relax, the muscle-driven wrinkles fade and muscle spasms are eliminated or greatly reduced. A Botox treatment typically lasts three to six months, because that's the amount of time it takes for the binding sites to recover and new nerve terminals to grow.

It's important to remember that Botox is not effective against all lines and wrinkles; it works only on "dynamic wrinkles," those that are accentuated by muscle movement. Those wrinkles include the three types listed here:

- Frown lines. The drug is injected into the area between the brows and causes the vertical wrinkles—those that cause the "furrowed brow look"—to relax, which also lifts the brow. This produces the effect of a more relaxed, less angry look.

- Horizontal forehead wrinkles. The muscles treated here are smaller than those between the brows, and they respond well to Botox. Injections along the forehead produce a smooth, younger-looking forehead.

- Crow's-feet. Nearly everyone who enjoys sun-worshiping (which causes squinting) and smiling can expect to have crow's-feet, and Botox can take them away by softening the lines on the outside of the eyes. There is a tendency for these wrinkles to reappear more quickly than those in other parts of the face, however, because other, untreated muscles near the eye that lift the corners of the mouth during smiling cannot be treated and so cause some secondary wrinkling of the skin around and under the eyes.

Other areas that are often treated with Botox but are less responsive because the wrinkles may be more related to sun damage (photo damage) and aging than to muscle contractions include lipstick lines (around the lips), laugh lines, marionette lines, and neck lines. To correct these wrinkles, doctors often will recommend either another cosmetic procedure completely or complementing Botox injections with another approach to get the desired look. Some of these optional cosmetic procedures are discussed in chapter 9.

THE BOTOX BOOM

For more than ten years, Botox has been used not only for specific medical purposes, but also to remove lines and wrinkles. Use of Botox in both of these categories is expected to increase now that Botox has been approved by the FDA for cosmetic uses. As it turns out, serendipity lives on. Doctors and researchers continue to find even more uses for this toxin, from relieving the pain associated with tension headache and migraines, to treating hyperhidrosis, a condition that causes people to sweat excessively. All uses of Botox are likely to increase dramatically as studies bear out its effectiveness and FDA approval is obtained for what are now off-label indications.

In the next chapter, we look at the noncosmetic uses of Botox, both the FDA-approved and off-label uses, how these discoveries have changed the lives of tens of thousands of people, and how this toxin has the potential to improve the lives of millions more.

QUESTIONS AND ANSWERS

I know doctors are allowed to use a drug for an off-label use once it's been approved for another purpose. But are there any guidelines that doctors must follow when deciding whether to use a drug for uses not approved by the Food and Drug Administration?

When the FDA approves a new drug for commercial use, the drug's producer is required to include prescribing guidelines (called a package insert) for physicians. These guidelines spell out the conditions for which the drug has been approved and the dosages and administration qualifications that go along with them. These guidelines result from the stringent studies that were conducted before the product became available to the public. But they are only guidelines; they are not laws or requirements. Thereafter, doctors may use the drug at their discretion for various medical conditions and at dosages they believe are appropriate for their patients. An example is the use of baby aspirin by patients with heart disease.

Off-label uses for drugs make up a very large percentage of how drugs are prescribed and used in the United States. That means many people are getting relief for symptoms even though the FDA has not officially approved the way they are getting it. As we've discussed, many of the medical uses of Botox are the result of off-label prescriptions. Read about them in chapter 5.

I'm not sure I'm comfortable having a poison injected into my body, even though it's highly diluted and everyone says it's safe. Is it possible to get a deadly dose of the drug? What is the lethal dose of Botox?

Like all drugs, Botox was tested thoroughly before it was approved by the Food and Drug Administration for human use. To determine a deadly dose of a drug for humans, animal studies are conducted. For Botox, animal studies suggest that the median human lethal dose is about 300 vials (or 30,000 units of Botox, because one vial contains 100 units) of *ingested,* not *injected,* Botox. That means you would need to swallow 300 vials of Botox for it to be deadly.

However, both cosmetic and medical uses of Botox involve injections, not ingestion. Besides, the number of units injected for both uses is dramatically lower than 30,000. The average number of units used for cosmetic procedures is 15 to 35 units per treatment area, and up to 200 units per session. If you are given Botox for a medical condition, the doses given are usually 200 to 400 units per treatment, although occasionally some can be as high as 800 units. There are no reports of anyone ever receiving a deadly dose of Botox, nor has anyone ever contracted botulism from Botox treatments.

5

BEYOND BEAUTY:
OTHER USES FOR BOTOX

Years before botulinum toxin A, or Botox, was used to erase the wrinkles from the faces of men and women everywhere, it was being injected into the muscles of thousands of people who suffered from painful, distressing, and often debilitating medical conditions. It was only by chance and good luck that researchers noted the cosmetic benefits.

But the fact that this extremely poisonous substance has the potential to provide safe, effective medical advantages is of great interest to those who can benefit from it. Some of those people include the millions who suffer from migraine, lower back pain, crossed-eyes (strabismus), and post-stroke spasticity, an inability to control muscle spasms, which is a condition experienced by many stroke patients. While these conditions (and many others that we discuss below) may appear to be unrelated, to some degree they all involve the muscles. They also are all conditions for which many people are finally getting significant help with Botox.

This chapter explores the medical uses of Botox and explains how it has the potential to provide relief and comfort to millions of people. Although not all of the uses discussed in this chapter have the approval of the Food and Drug Administration, many doctors are using Botox for off-label uses, such as for migraine and lower back pain. Whether FDA-approved or off-label, Botox is providing some much-needed help to many people.

MIGRAINE AND OTHER HEADACHE PAIN

Much of what we discover about new treatments and medications is the result of serendipity. This was the case with Botox and headache pain. When doctors who were giving Botox injections for wrinkles began to get reports from their patients that they were also getting relief from all types of headache pain, including migraine and tension headaches, they listened.

Doctors began to share their patients' stories with their colleagues at meetings and conferences. Patients also told their friends about the relief they were getting. As the anecdotal stories began to pile up, it became apparent that scientific investigations were needed to validate this spreading phenomenon, especially given that migraine and tension headaches are both very common, debilitating, and expensive health problems in the United States. Migraine, usually the more severe of the two types, affects an estimated 28 million Americans, according to the National Institute of Neurological Disorders and Stroke. Seventy-five percent of those affected are women. Migraine takes a significant toll not only on those who experience the pain but on the U.S. economy as well: it costs Americans about $13 billion in lost work and productivity every year.

More than 78 percent of Americans experience chronic or bouts of tension headache during their lifetime. Forty-four percent of them say that the pain can limit their ability to function. Finding an effective way to relieve these painful conditions would be a welcome discovery to many.

At the Thomas Jefferson University School of Medicine in Philadelphia, researchers studied 123 patients who had a history of migraine. They found that when they injected Botox into the foreheads of migraine sufferers, the patients experienced a significant decline in the frequency and severity of their migraines, as well as a reduction in vomiting, a common side effect of migraine.

· At the University of Toronto, doctors compared two groups of patients who were experiencing headache associated with neck pain. Some of the patients received injections of Botox in their neck and head, while others received a placebo (an inactive substance given to some participants in a study so researchers can measure the effects of the active treatment compared to no treatment). Four weeks after the injections, those who had received the Botox had significantly greater range of neck movement and elimination or reduction of pain when compared with the placebo group, who had no change.

Researchers at the St. Louis University School of Medicine in Missouri found that in most patients they treated, small doses of Botox relaxed the muscles that trigger or perpetuate tension headache pain. After receiving eight low-dose injections along the forehead—similar to those given to treat forehead wrinkles—patients reported relief for up to three months. That relief came in the form of a significant decrease in intensity of pain and frequency of headaches. They also reported that those symptoms that did occur were easier to control with medication.

Other studies, both here and abroad, continue to substantiate the claims that Botox is effective in both treating and preventing migraine and in the treatment of tension headaches and the less common, but severe, cluster headaches. So far, most studies of the use of Botox for migraine and tension headache pain have found that 25 units, which is about the same amount given to remove forehead wrinkles, is effective in preventing or relieving pain. Some studies have used injections of up to 80 units per treatment.

However, not everyone who has migraine or tension headaches is a candidate for Botox injections, says Ghazala Hayat, MD, associate professor of neurology at St. Louis University School of Medicine. At least for now, only those who have not responded well to other treatment medications should be considered. Because of the cost of Botox, insurance companies generally won't cover the injections unless all other treatments have failed.

Eleanor's Story

Eleanor, a twenty-eight-year-old marketing analyst, knows the benefits of one of the off-label uses of Botox. For more than a decade, she suffered from migraines, severe head pain that attacked her about every six to eight weeks.

"The pain sent me straight to bed," she recalls. "Most of the time I was sick to my stomach as well. I usually lost at least one day's work, sometimes two. My boss was very understanding, but the pain disrupted every part of my life. I tried different medications, including sumatriptan, and even the herb feverfew, but none of them helped enough to allow me to do more than the simplest things. I really wanted to find a way to at least reduce the severity of the migraines so that I could live a reasonably better life."

When a friend told Eleanor about reading that some doctors were injecting Botox into the foreheads of people who have migraine or tension headaches, she immediately called her neurologist. Eleanor's doctor had heard about Botox but had not given the injections, so he made a few phone calls and finally referred her to a colleague who had been using Botox successfully in some of his migraine patients.

Eleanor made an appointment and got her first injection six weeks after a recent migraine attack. Then she waited, and waited, and four months later she still had not had another migraine. "It was wonderful," she says. "And when I did have another attack, at five months after the injection, it was much less severe than I was used to having."

EXCESSIVE SWEATING

Excessive sweating, or hyperhidrosis, is a problem suffered by up to 1 percent of adults in the United States, according to the American Academy of Dermatology, and many cases go unreported. In some people it is caused by overactive nerves that keep sending messages to the sweat glands to produce more perspiration. It can also be a symptom of another condition, such as an overactive thyroid or nerve damage from diabetes. In other cases, the cause is unknown.

The human body has more than five million sweat glands, and people who have hyperhidrosis are well aware of the embarrassment and discomfort they can cause. These individuals can literally sweat through their clothes in a matter of minutes. They often spend thousands of dollars on dry cleaning and purchasing new clothes to replace those that they ruin.

"My excessive sweating was a constant source of embarrassment and anxiety for me," says Ron, a thirty-year-old patent attorney. "My hands would get so wet I had to always make sure I wiped them off on a handkerchief I kept in my pocket or briefcase before I shook someone's hand. I was always afraid to meet clients. I avoided social situations whenever possible. I was willing to do anything to eliminate the problem, and then I heard about Botox. Getting those injections has made a big difference in my life. I feel confident again. I'm not afraid to meet people and shake hands. It has meant a lot for my career and my life in general."

In 1994, researchers discovered that Botox injections could significantly reduce excessive sweating. Today, injections of Botox are given to decrease sweating on the palms, underarms, soles of the feet, forehead, and genital region, although the first two areas mentioned are the most common ones treated. The toxin blocks the release of acetycholine, the chemical responsible for stimulating the sweat glands.

Compared with the amount of Botox given to eliminate wrinkles (typically around 25 units), the amount injected to stop excessive sweating may be eight times that amount. In a study done in Germany, researchers found that injecting 200 units of the drug per armpit resulted in up to 19 months of relatively sweat-free living for about half of the patients they treated. The range of sweat-free time enjoyed by the patients was 12 to 29 months.

Another German study found that for patients who received 200 units of Botox per palm, sweaty palms were eliminated for an average of 12 months, and even up to 22 months in some patients. The researchers also report that giving 200 units is just as safe as giving a lower dose, but you can expect to enjoy a longer sweat-free period with the higher dose.

Leslie Baumann, MD, director of cosmetic dermatology at the University of Miami Medical School, has treated hundreds of people who have this condition. When treating the palms, she notes that "although some patients complain about a loss of muscle strength, the change is not detectable using a dynamometer, which measures handgrip strength. I have found that it only bothers tennis players, weight lifters, and pianists. Overall, the treatments work really well and are life-changing for many patients." Injecting into the palms is painful, however, so many doctors use nerve blocks to numb the hands. Some studies have reported that patients treated in their palms have experienced fever, mild loss of fingertip sensation, and headache after their treatments.

Dr. Baumann also reports that injections into the armpit work very well and are much less painful than treating the palms. She has not encountered any side effects when injecting into the armpit. Similar results can be expected from injections in the genital/groin area.

Sometimes Botox is used to eliminate sweating for more cosmetic reasons. Some celebrities reportedly visit their doctors for Botox injections before movie openings, awards ceremonies, and other big social events so they won't sweat in public. Many of these stars don't have hyperhidrosis, just a case of not wanting to ruin dresses and suits that can cost tens of thousands of dollars, or not wanting to drop their Tony or Oscar when they go up on stage. Most people, however, would probably find the $500 to $1,500 price tag per treatment area for this nonmedical procedure to be an unaffordable luxury.

BACK PAIN

Back pain is one of the most common and debilitating health problems in the United States, and it is also one of the most frustrating conditions to treat. Nearly 90 percent of adults in American can expect to experience back pain—most often lower back pain—during their lifetime. Chronic back pain hurts in another way too: it costs the American economy about $50 billion a year in medical costs and lost earnings.

In a study conducted at Walter Reed Army Medical Center in Washington, DC, and published in 2001 in *Neurology,* researchers reported that injections of Botox provided significant relief of chronic lower back pain. Three weeks after treatment, 73 percent of patients who received Botox reported greater than 50 percent pain relief, compared with only 25 percent of patients who had received a placebo. Eight weeks after they had received their injections, 60 percent of the treated patients and less than 13 percent of the placebo patients reported having at least 50 percent pain relief.

There are two reasons why Botox may help with back pain, says Dr. Hayat. When the drug is administered properly, it can cause temporary muscle weakness, which blocks the ability of the muscle to contract or stay in spasm. Such spasms are often the cause of an individual's lower back pain.

There is also some evidence that Botox may directly address pain by having an impact on pain receptors. It's still too soon to know if this is true, but if it is, it could mean that Botox could help other painful conditions that do not necessarily involve the muscles.

Side effects of Botox injections for back pain may include nausea, pain at the injection site, and dizziness. Botox injections are usually reserved for people who have not responded to other types of pain medications or treatments for their back pain. Administration of Botox for back pain is an off-label use.

OTHER PAINFUL CONDITIONS

Uses for Botox injections in the treatment of pain continue to grow as researchers conduct further studies. Here are a few more conditions for which you may want to consider Botox injections.

Myofascial Pain Syndrome

Myofascial pain syndrome is a common although poorly understood condition in which trigger points—taut bands of muscle fibers—are tender and twitch involuntarily when touched. These trigger points, which can appear at various places on the body, can cause referred pain, pain that emerges elsewhere in the body from where pressure is placed. Pressure to a trigger point on the lower back, for example, may send pain down the leg.

Studies show that injections of Botox are more effective and longer lasting than conventional steroid treatment when it comes to relieving pain in myofascial pain syndrome. In a study conducted at the Pain Evaluation and Treatment Center in Tulsa, Oklahoma, 70 percent of patients with the painful syndrome in their back and extremities who received injections over two years had good to excellent pain relief that lasted for an average of 2.5 to 3.6 months. Relief from symptoms typically occurred within seven days of injection. After one year, 10 percent of the patients had no pain at all. Because the patients experienced significant pain relief, they were better able to tolerate more aggressive therapeutic exercises and enjoy a better quality of life.

Fibromyalgia

Myofascial pain syndrome is often confused with fibromyalgia, a condition that also has tender trigger points, but ones that do not cause a twitch response. Fibromyalgia is characterized by muscle pain, depression, fatigue, and interrupted sleep patterns. The majority of its victims are women, usually between the ages of thirty and fifty. The American College of Rheumatology estimates that 3 to 6 million Americans have the disorder, the cause of which is unknown.

Both myofascial pain syndrome and fibromyalgia are being treated with Botox as an off-label use by some doctors, and trials are being conducted at several institutions. Rheumatologists who have given injections of Botox for fibromyalgia report that the drug takes effect after about a week, and that patients experience relief for about three to four months before needing another injection.

Sciatica

Sciatica is the often severe pain that travels down from one side of the buttocks along the sciatic nerve, which is the largest nerve in the body. The pain runs along the back of the leg, often extending to the foot. The pain can begin suddenly or come on gradually, and it typically gets worse the more the affected leg is moved. It is usually described as a sharp, shooting, stabbing, or even burning pain, and can last a few days or even months. Numbness can occur in the leg as well.

At Louisiana State University in Shreveport, patients with sciatic pain who received Botox injections reported significant relief from their pain. Three months after receiving their injections, 48 of 50 patients had a decrease in pain of 45 percent or more. In Europe, Botox has proven effective in the treatment of long-term sciatic pain. Additional studies are needed of this off-label use of Botox.

Whiplash

Another common painful condition is whiplash, which is usually associated with motor vehicle accidents. At the University of Toronto, patients who had whiplash-associated disorder due to an automobile accident were treated with Botox. Half of the 26 patients received 100 units of Botox, while the other half received a placebo. One month after the injection, the treated patients had significant improvement in pain and in range of motion, while the placebo patients benefited from no such change.

POST-STROKE SPASTICITY

Many stroke patients experience what is called post-stroke spasticity, a condition in which a muscle does not respond to the signals sent to it by the nervous system. As a result, the muscle remains contracted, or clenched, which causes pain and restricts movement and the ability to perform daily tasks like eating and dressing. The arms are affected more often than the legs, and it is common to see an arm of a stroke patient being held close or tight to the chest.

Researchers have found that injections of Botox into the contracted muscles can block the signals that cause the muscles to contract, thus allowing the muscles to relax and giving patients better function and mobility. At Indiana University, investigators studied 91 patients who had post-stroke spasticity. Patients were randomly chosen to receive either 90, 180, or 360 units of the toxin or a placebo. After a few weeks, patients who had received Botox had a decrease in spasticity compared with patients who had received a placebo. Patients who received the highest dose of the drug had the most relief.

Each treatment can provide relief from spasticity for three to six months before the effects wear off. Side effects are mild and can include swelling or soreness at the injection site, fatigue, headache, dizziness, and excess muscle weakness. Although a small percentage of patients do not respond to the injections, up to 97 percent of them can expect at least partial relief from spasticity.

Canada has approved the use of Botox for treatment of spasticity in stroke patients, but the Food and Drug Administration has not given approval for such use in the United States. Some doctors are giving Botox for spasticity as an off-label use to help improve the lives of patients who have had a stroke.

One of the biggest frustrations for Margaret after her stroke was her inability to unclench her right fist and arm and do normal, everyday things like getting dressed and feeding herself. "I hated having to depend on other people to help me with simple things," says the sixty-eight-year-old retired teacher. "I was used to being independent, but this stroke took a lot of that away. I wanted to be able to regain at least some of my mobility so I could care for myself as much as possible."

Fortunately for Margaret, she entered a rehabilitation facility where Botox was used. The injections have helped her with her therapy and in learning how to live with her limitations.

Dr. Hayat would like to see more stroke patients have the opportunity to experience the benefits of Botox. "The best time to treat them is within the first few months of their stroke," she says. "When it's used during rehabilitation, it helps patients relax and so they can better do and benefit from their therapy."

CEREBRAL PALSY

Cerebral palsy is a term used to describe a permanent condition in which there has been damage to the cerebrum of the brain, resulting in disorders in movement and posture. Exactly what causes this damage is not always known, but possible culprits include lack of oxygen to the brain during delivery, low blood-sugar levels, injury to the brain during birth, exposure to certain infections during pregnancy (for example, rubeola and German measles), and jaundice.

Cerebral palsy is the most common cause of disability in children, and occurs in approximately one in 400 live births. Slightly more males than females are affected, and it appears more often in premature infants and in those with a low birth weight.

Botox injections, which are an off-label use for this condition, have proven very helpful in relieving some of the symptoms of the disease. The drug is effective in relieving toe-
walking (an inability to place the heel flat on the ground), a
common feature of children who have cerebral palsy, and
muscle spasms. The injections are given to the specific leg
muscles that are affected by the disease, and the toxin stops
the messages that travel from the nerve to the affected muscle, telling it to contract. The drug allows therapists to then
stretch the relaxed muscles and stimulate their normal
growth. Stretching the muscles allows the children to walk
more normally and to gain better balance, and it also reduces
spasticity.

Botox injections are usually effective for up to six months,
at which point they need to be repeated. The drug is most effective when it is given during the early stages of the disease,
when the child's bones are still growing and before any bone
deformity can develop.

STRABISMUS

You probably know this condition better as crossed eyes, a vision problem in which a person cannot voluntarily align both
eyes at the same time under normal conditions. One or both
eyes may be turned up, down, toward the nose, or to the side,
and this condition may always be present or occur intermit-
tently. When it isn't constant, the cause may be stress or illness.

About 5 percent of children have some degree of strabismus, and contrary to what some people think, it is not a condition that children usually outgrow. Adults who have
strabismus have either had the condition since childhood, or

acquired it from an injury or illness as an adult. Strabismus affects about 4 percent of adults.

Having one or both eyes misaligned is not only a vision problem (double vision is common), but it also can make people embarrassed and uncomfortable in social settings and other areas of their lives. Many people who have strabismus experience limited job and career opportunities, not because they aren't capable, but because they may be discriminated against based on how they look. They also often lack self-confidence and self-esteem.

"Having strabismus has always made it hard for me to feel confident when I'm around a lot of people," says Melissa, a twenty-four-year-old graduate student. "I've always felt self-conscious with men, and I haven't done much dating because of my eyes. Wearing dark glasses helps, but you have to take them off eventually!"

Melissa did some research about the use of Botox and found an ophthalmologist who was treating patients who have strabismus. She went for a consultation and decided to give it a try. Although she was nervous about having an injection, she says the drops of local anesthetic and decongestant the doctor gave her a few minutes before the injection made the whole experience bearable. About two weeks after her injection, she returned to the doctor for an assessment.

"I feel as if it's changed my life," she says. "I don't feel as if everyone is staring at me anymore. Right now I work in the university lab, but I'll be looking for a regular full-time job soon. Before I had the injections, I worried about going on interviews. Now I feel more confident."

The Food and Drug Administration approved Botox for treatment of strabismus in 1989 for people aged twelve years and older. Botox injections can be an alternative to surgery for people who have strabismus. The injections are done in the doctor's office and need to be given about every six months, depending on how the individual responds.

BLEPHAROSPASM

This eye condition, which can affect one or both eyes, causes the eyelids to spasm closed, uncontrollably and repeatedly. Occasionally the spasms also appear in the neck or face. Blepharospasm usually first appears among people who are in their fifties or sixties, and it affects women more often than men. About 300 out of every one million people have the disease.

The first symptom of blepharospasm is usually uncontrollable blinking, leading up to a time when the eyelids simply refuse to remain open. Thus, individuals with this disorder are essentially blind, even though they have the ability to see.

The exact cause of blepharospasm is not known, but it seems to be the result of communication problems in the area of the brain that is responsible for controlling the eyelid muscles (orbicularis oculi). The symptoms are often triggered by fatigue and emotional stress. Bright lights, watching television, and driving often make the condition worse.

Injections of botulinum toxin A (brand name Oculinum, the ocular form of Botox) are often the first treatment used for blepharospasm. The toxin is injected into the upper and lower eyelids of the involved eye, and results are usually apparent in one to fourteen days. Repeat injections are needed every three to six months, depending on how severe the condition is. Side effects may include drooping of the eye (in

about 10 percent of patients this problem resolves spontaneously within two weeks), blurred vision, eye tearing, and
local bleeding.

Not everyone responds to botulinum injections, however.
For those individuals, surgery (cutting the involved muscles)
may decrease the spasms. Surgery may also need to be an option for people who have received botulinum injections for
many years, as they can build up an immunity to the drug,
which means it's no longer effective for them. The FDA approved the use of botulinum toxin A for blepharospasm in
1989.

SPASMODIC TORTICOLLIS
(CERVICAL DYSTONIA)

Spasmodic torticollis ("torti" is Latin for "twisted"; "collis"
means "neck") is a disorder in which painful muscle spasms
occur in the neck and force the head to turn to one side, although they can also cause the head to be pulled forward or
backward as well. It is the most common type of dystonia, a
category of disorders characterized by abnormal, impaired
muscle tone and movements. (The second most common type
of dystonia is blepharospasm.)

Spasmodic torticollis affects approximately 3 out of every
10,000 people and usually appears in people ages 30 to 60.
More than 83,000 people in the United States have this condition. The FDA approved Botox for treatment of this dystonia in December 2000.

Spasmodic torticollis does not affect other areas of the
body, but the forceful neck movements can severely limit a
person's ability to function. Although the cause is unknown,

experts believe the originating point is in the lower part of the brain, from which signals are sent that cause an abnormal contraction of the muscles in the neck. Injections of Botox interrupt these signals, allowing the muscles to relax and the head and neck to remain unaffected. Botox is not a cure, however, and the effect of the toxin wears off in about 3 to 4 months. Thus, repeat injections are needed to control the spasms. Approximately 75 to 85 percent of patients get some relief of pain and spasms beginning three to five days after receiving the injections.

Side effects from the injections into the neck can include pain or bruising at the injection site, headache, and new pain in the neck muscles, which usually disappears after 1 to 3 weeks. Up to one-third of patients experience swallowing problems beginning 3 to 10 days after receiving the injection. This problem usually lasts for 1 to 3 weeks. Patients report feeling as if food is caught in their throat, and when they eat, they must swallow several times for food to clear the throat.

Weakness of the neck muscles is another common problem. This side effect typically appears about two weeks after the injection and can last for several weeks. It's noticed most often when people get out of bed or when they lean forward. In rare cases, people develop resistance to the toxin, which means that after they receive several treatments, the injections are no longer as effective. Frequent injections or high doses of Botox seem to predispose people to resistance. For this reason, doctors typically give the lowest dose that will produce the best effect and adminster treatments no more frequently than every two to three months.

OTHER DYSTONIAS

Several other types of dystonia, although less common than blepharospasm and cervical dystonia, also respond to Botox. Hemifacial spasm is a painful and often embarrassing condition that involves the sudden, simultaneous contraction of the muscles on one side of the face. The spasm may last for only a second or for several seconds, and it can recur several times a day. Often, a hemifacial spasm is caused by a blood vessel that is pressing against the facial nerve, which travels from the brain to the facial muscles, or it can be caused by a tumor within the brain. Botox injections are an effective treatment when the cause cannot be found and the possibility of a brain tumor has been ruled out, or when the doctors decide that the condition cannot be treated using surgery or oral medications. Botox was approved for the treatment of hemifacial spasm by the FDA in 1989.

Oromandibular dystonia is characterized by continuous spasms of the muscles on both sides of the face as well as the neck, tongue, and larynx. In severe cases, it also affects the breathing muscles. Because of the severity of this condition, Botox injections are usually used along with other medications to get relief.

People who have spasmodic dysphonia experience sudden interruptions to their speech when their laryngeal muscles (the vocal cords) spasm. Botox has proven effective in significantly reducing the symptoms and allowing people to speak fluently again. Injections are typically needed up to every six months.

OTHER MEDICAL USES FOR BOTOX

One of the most recently reported (May 2002) medical uses for Botox is for overactive bladder. More than 17 million Americans suffer from this condition, which is characterized by the need to urinate more than eight times within a 24-hour period, an immediate and strong urge to urinate, and incontinence, which is an inability to stop the urge to urinate, resulting in leakage of urine. Overactive bladder can significantly affect the quality of a person's life, and be the cause of great embarrassment. Many people are so embarrassed that they don't even seek help for it: an estimated 80 percent of people remain untreated for this problem.

Many of these people may find relief with Botox. That's because overactive bladder is caused by the involuntary contractions of a muscle (detrusor muscle) that controls the bladder. Injections of Botox can help stop the contractions, which allows the bladder to function normally.

This was the case at the University of Pittsburgh School of Medicine, where researchers treated 50 people who had overactive bladder. Forty-one of the 50 patients reported that their incontinence stopped completely or decreased within seven days of receiving Botox injections. The results lasted for approximately six months.

Researchers continue to find more medical conditions that frequently respond to Botox injections. So far, only a limited number of studies have been done, but many of the results are promising. Some of those conditions not already mentioned include multiple sclerosis (a debilitating central nervous system disease); Parkinson's disease (foot dystonia is seen in about one-third of patients who have been taking oral medications for three years or more); temporomandibular disorder (TMD), a painful condition that affects the jaw and face muscles; and writer's cramp (a hand dystonia), in which there are involuntary muscle contractions in the wrist, fingers, and sometimes the forearm.

HOW TO GET BOTOX FOR MEDICAL USES

If you are like the majority of people, you have never heard about the medical uses of Botox before now. Yet the day may come when you or a loved one may want to consider Botox to relieve the pain and discomfort associated with a medical condition like one of those discussed in this chapter. Dr. Hayat, who has been using Botox for more than fourteen years for various medical disorders, is hopeful that information about the medical uses of Botox will begin to reach the general population and the people who really need it. "I'm sure that in the next five to ten years, we'll have many more physicians familiar with and using Botox for medical reasons," she says.

If you or someone you know is experiencing any of the conditions discussed in this chapter, and conventional treatments have not provided meaningful relief, talk to your doctor about Botox. If your doctor cannot help you, ask if he or she can refer you to someone who can. You may also contact your local hospital referral service, or one of the organizations listed in the Appendix that deals with the specific condition you need to treat. Relief may be little more than a telephone call away.

A final note: It will probably be difficult to convince your insurance carrier to cover Botox injections for medical conditions that require off-label (non-FDA-approved) uses, such as for migraine or back pain. If you are not prepared to pay for Botox treatment out of pocket, talk to your doctor and insurance company before undergoing treatment to determine if your treatments will be covered.

QUESTIONS AND ANSWERS

I've been suffering with terrible migraines for more than ten years. My doctor has never mentioned Botox to me. Where can I get treated?

First, talk to your doctor and see if he or she can refer you to a physician who is familiar with treating migraine with Botox. If you cannot get a referral, you can contact your local hospital's physician referral service. Organizations that may help you locate a physician who deals with Botox include the American Council for Headache Education and the American Chronic Pain Association. Contact information for these organizations is in the Appendix.

My ten-year-old daughter has crossed eyes. Is she too young to get Botox?

The FDA has approved Botox for treatment of strabismus in people aged twelve years and older. For children younger than twelve it is considered an off-label use. Talk to your doctor about having your daughter treated by an ophthalmologist who has experience with Botox.

My son was diagnosed with cerebral palsy recently, and my doctor hasn't mentioned using Botox. Should I ask him about it?

Certainly. It's possible he or she is not familiar with using it, or is not aware of the studies that are ongoing. In the fast-changing world of medicine, it's very difficult for doctors to stay abreast of all the latest developments. Also, Botox is not indicated in every case of cerebral palsy, so it may not be indicated for your son. The best response is usually seen in children younger than six years of age who have not developed joints that are fixed and rigid. Botox is most helpful when it is given during the early phase of spasticity, before a child's bones have fully developed and before any bone abnormalities have formed.

For more information, you can contact the United Cerebral Palsy Research Foundation at 1-800-872-5827, or your local United Cerebral Palsy branch office.

I will be getting Botox injections for my chronic lower back pain, and my doctor mentioned that he will use an EMG. What is an EMG?

Physicians sometimes use an electromyogram (EMG) to help guide the injections of Botox. An EMG has a hollow needle that helps the doctor locate the area of the affected muscles that are experiencing the worst contractions. Once that site is located, he can inject the drug, thus helping ensure the best results. An EMG is often used when Botox is given for medical uses. Physicians who use Botox to eliminate wrinkles in the neck often use it as well.

I don't think I have hyperhidrosis, but I do sweat a great deal when I'm very nervous. I have to give a big lecture next month, and I'd like to look cool and confident. Should I get Botox injections?

Some celebrities line up for Botox injections before award

ceremonies and galas so they won't sweat in public. However, you may want to reconsider when you learn that Botox injections for hyperhidrosis normally run about $700 to $1,500, depending on the areas treated and the amount of Botox used. That's $350 to $700 per armpit, palm, and so on. Talk to your doctor about your concerns regarding excessive sweating. You should be evaluated to see if you do have hyperhidrosis and if a medical condition is its cause.

I'd like to talk to my doctor about getting Botox injections for my migraines. Will the injections be covered by insurance?

Botox is not approved by the FDA for the treatment of migraine, and when the injections are used for such off-label medical purposes, they are often not covered by insurance plans. You will generally have to pay for such treatment out of pocket. In most cases, insurance does cover injections used to treat strabismus, blepharospasm, hemifacial spasm, and cervical dystonia. Botox for cosmetic purposes is not covered by insurance plans.

6

FINDING THE RIGHT DOCTOR

FINDING THE RIGHT DOCTOR for any type of health or medical issue requires careful thought and planning. The person you choose will be guiding you through decisions, treatments, and procedures that can have a significant impact on your health and quality of life. Such careful consideration also applies when you are choosing the right physician to perform your Botox injections plus any other cosmetic procedures you may want.

Katrina is a no-nonsense woman; just ask anyone who knows her. "When I set out to do something, I explore all my options and all the avenues," she says. "When I go to a doctor, I've done my homework before I even step into the office. I know about the doctor and the practice, and I've read up on the latest information about the condition I'm considering, and I've checked out the drugs that might be prescribed."

So when it came time for Katrina to consider Botox injections, she was her usual meticulous self. "I read all the literature and articles I could find. I talked to some people who had had the injections. And then I started to look around for the right doctor."

When it comes to getting Botox injections, Debra Jaliman, MD, a clinical instructor at Mount Sinai School of Medicine and a dermatologist in private practice in New York City, tells people to look for one of four different professionals: "We believe a dermatologist, a plastic surgeon, a cosmetic ear-nose-throat [otorhinolaryngologist] doctor, or a cosmetic ophthalmologist are the people qualified to give these injections," she says. (See below, "Who's Qualified and Why.")

However, other physicians, including general practitioners, and even nurse practitioners are giving cosmetic injections to unsuspecting patients. Although doctors with specialties other than those named by Dr. Jaliman know how to give injections, Botox treatments require more than just knowing how to give a shot.

Who's Qualified and Why

If you're looking for a qualified professional to administer your Botox injections, and to discuss and perform other cosmetic procedures with you, it's best to choose a doctor from one of the following specialty areas. That's not to say that an internist or an obstetrician doesn't know how to give an injection. However, chances are these professionals aren't intimately familiar with skin conditions, facial musculature, and facial aesthetic enhancement. Also they probably don't fully appreciate the art of cosmetic rejuvenation and how to reshape a person's face.

Dermatologist and Dermatologic Surgeon. Dermatologists specialize in the diagnosis and treatment, medical and surgical, of disorders that affect the hair, nails, and skin, such as acne, wrinkles, scars, age spots, and hair loss. Once they complete their four years of medical school and one to three years of postgraduate training, they complete three years of dermatology residency. Some dermatologists choose to specialize in surgical and cosmetic dermatology, and complete another year or two of fellowship training in dermatologic surgery. Dermatologic surgery training focuses on procedures that are usually office based and includes skin cancer removal and various cosmetic procedures from Botox and soft-tissue augmentation to chemical peels, laser surgery, and liposuction. Look for a dermatologist who specializes in the procedures in which you are interested. The American Society for Dermatologic Surgery website www.aboutskinsurgery.com can guide you.

Ophthalmologist. These physicians are trained in both the medical and the surgical treatment of the eye. Not all ophthalmologists are qualified to do Botox injections or cosmetic procedures, however. Those who subspecialize in cosmetic eye surgery are often referred to as occuplastic surgeons. They often perform eyelid surgery to reduce wrinkles and to eliminate drooping upper and lower eyelids.

Otorhinolaryngologist (Ear, Nose, and Throat Surgeon). Also known as ENT doctors, these professionals specialize in surgical procedures on the ear, nose, throat, and face. If you are considering an ENT for Botox or other cosmetic procedures, look for one who is a member of the American Academy of Facial Plastic and Reconstructive Surgery. Members of this organization must have completed at least four to six years of special training. ENT doctors are also referred to as facial plastic surgeons.

Plastic Surgeon. Doctors who specialize in the reconstruction and repair of the external body and face are called plastic surgeons. Board-certified plastic surgeons must undergo at least five to six years of approved residency training.

Within the category of plastic surgeons there are subspecialties. Surgeons who focus on repairing injuries or birth defects are usually known as reconstructive plastic surgeons, while those who concentrate on the enhancement of one's appearance are called aesthetic plastic surgeons. Naturally, if you're interested in a cosmetic procedure, you should consider a doctor in the latter group.

The Bottom Line: Any doctor you choose for any treatment should be board-certified in his or her area.

The problem is, says Dr. Jaliman, the general public sees Botox injection as being a deceptively simple procedure, but it really isn't simple at all. It requires a specialist who is intimately familiar with handling skin and the problems related to it, as well as conditions associated with the muscles that control facial expression. Simply knowing how to give an injection is definitely not enough qualification.

Dr. Jaliman explains that the doctor you go to should be

experienced in knowing how much Botox to give in order to achieve a pleasing look. "Some people don't want any facial expression," she explains. "They want what I call the 'Stepford wife' look. But others want facial expression, so we do what I call 'Botox light,' which means I give less toxin. That's why I consider this a real art. Botox is not just about paralyzing or not paralyzing certain muscles. Sometimes you may just want to weaken them."

Looking for the Right Doctor

When choosing someone to reshape your face, you'll want to make sure he or she is not only well qualified but is also caring and conservative. Here are some places for you to search.

www.botox.com. A good place to start is the website developed by Allergan, the manufacturer of Botox. This Internet site lists all the doctors, by their specialties, who have been trained in the administration of Botox.

Friends. When it comes to cosmetic procedures, friends, family members, and others with whom you have a good, trusting relationship can be your best source for referrals. Firsthand experience is the best: if your cousin says she has a friend who was "very happy with Dr. X" but you don't know that friend, you may want to disregard that referral. Talk directly to people who have had Botox injections, or any other procedure you are considering. Naturally, your friends won't have all the information you need, so you'll still need to consult other sources.

Your Family Doctor. If you have a trusted family physician, you may ask her or him for referrals. If your doctor gives you a name or two, ask if your doctor has seen the work of these specialists and how long he or she has known them. If your doctor gives you only one name, ask for at least one more in case you want to get a second opinion.

Hospital Referral. Hospitals maintain a referral list of physicians who are associated with each specific hospital. Typically, university teaching hospitals are more selective when choosing doctors for their staff. You can obtain a hospital's referral list by calling the hospital's main number and asking for the referral service. Of course, you'll only get a list of doctors who practice at that particular hospital, so your choice is limited.

Where Not to Look: Botox Parties.

You've probably heard about Botox parties: where doctors (or sometimes nonphysicians) invite people to their office to socialize, enjoy some refreshments, and line up for their Botox injections. Dermatologist Ronald Fragen, MD, of Fragen Cosmetic Surgery Center in Palm Springs, California, urges people to think before they sign up for one of these parties. "While getting your Botox injections at a social gathering may sound cute, do you *really* want to receive your medical treatment at a cocktail party?"

Leslie Baumann, MD, director of cosmetic dermatology at the University of Miami Medical School and a participant in the FDA trials for Botox, also warns consumers about Botox parties. "I know of no reputable physicians who hold these parties," she says. "The American Academy of Dermatology, the American Society for Dermatologic Surgery, and the company that makes Botox have all come out with written statements against these parties. You should question the motives of any physician who engages in these unprofessional events."

Make a List, Check It Twice

After consulting these sources, you should gather two or three names of prospective physicians. Now you want to meet each of them and find out whether they meet your criteria. To help you do that, we've compiled a list of questions you should consider when screening your candidates.

If all of this sounds a bit intense to you, remember that you plan to have a long-term relationship with the doctor you ultimately choose. While you may only want Botox injections now, sometime in the future you might want to add other procedures, such as laser resurfacing or collagen injections. If you already have a doctor whom you trust and who knows you and your face well, think how much more comfortable and confident you'll feel when you're ready to have the other cosmetic procedures.

Edie remembers how her sister thought Edie was being overly cautious when she went shopping for a Botox doc. "She told me that getting Botox injections was no big deal, and so why was I being so picky," says Edie. "Yet my sister had just picked someone out of the phone book, someone who wasn't really qualified to give the injections, and she ended up with a droopy eyelid. Sure, it went away after a few months, but she was pretty upset the entire time. After that, she asked me for the name of *my* doctor!"

Edie narrowed down her list of three candidates to one by first meeting with each of them and asking her list of questions, as well as making observations about the office staff and the office itself. Make sure to take this list with you on your interview so you don't forget anything.

Questions for the Doctor

- What are the doctor's credentials? Is the doctor board-certified in dermatology or in another appropriate area? Do not be afraid to ask to see credentials. The doctor may have a website where this information can be accessed easily, or you could speak with the practice manager if you prefer not to ask the doctor directly. However, if the doctor is offended or refuses, you know you have the wrong doctor. You can also check to see if doctors have had any malpractice suits against them, or if they have been disciplined. See "Checking Out Your Doctor" on the following page.

- How many Botox patients has the doctor treated? While it's hard to place an exact figure on how many procedures is "enough," you probably want a doctor who has done at least 50 or has had formal training. Also, ask to see before-and-after pictures of the patients he or she has treated. Many doctors now keep before-and-after shots on their computers for prospective patients to view. You can also ask for the names of patients who have had the treatments so you can ask them questions.

- How did the doctor receive his or her training in Botox injections? Some clinicians learn about Botox injections from preceptorships, in which experts in Botox teach doctors about injection techniques, the appropriate sites for injection, and how to handle the toxin. The manufacturer of Botox, Allergan, Inc., provides instruction for qualified doctors, including dermatologists, plastic surgeons, cosmetic ear-nose-throat doctors, and cosmetic ophthalmologists. Their website www.botox.com

lists the national training preceptors. Instruction is also provided by the American Academy of Dermatology.

- What results can you expect? No one can absolutely guarantee specific results, but the doctor should be able to tell you, based on experience, how you will look once the Botox takes effect. The same is true of any other cosmetic procedure you may be looking into.

- What complications are possible? Side effects of Botox injections and any other procedures you are considering should be explained to you fully.

- What is the cost? The cost of Botox injections varies depending on the doctor. Some doctors charge by the unit of drug given; others charge by the area treated. Ask your doctor how he or she charges, and what the cost will be for the treatment you need. The average cost per treatment can range from $200 to $600, depending on the area treated and the part of the country in which you live. (See the discussion on "The Price of Botox" later in this chapter.)

Checking Out Your Doctor

If you want to find out whether a doctor is board-certified in his or her particular field, you can contact the appropriate organization listed here. The American Board of Medical Specialists can verify the board certification of any doctor among its twenty-four member organizations. Or you can contact the specific organization directly.

American Board of Medical Specialists
1007 Church Street, Suite 404
Evanston, IL 60201-5913
847-491-9091

American Board of Dermatology
1 Ford Place
Detroit, MI 48823-6319
313-874-1088

American Board of Ophthalmology
111 Presidential Blvd, Suite 241
Bala Cynwyd, PA 19004
610-664-1175

American Board of Otolaryngology
211 Norfolk, Suite 800
Houston, TX 77098-4044
713-528-6200

American Board of Plastic Surgery
Seven Penn Center, Suite 400
1635 Market Street
Philadelphia, PA 19103-2204
215-587-9322

You can also check the training and certification status of your candidates at the American Medical Association's Physician Select, an online service that is free to consumers. It is located at www.ama-assn.org/aps/amahg.htm. This service, however, does not provide information about any disciplinary action that may have been taken against a doctor.

If you would like to find out about any disciplinary action, including fraud, you can contact Medi-Net (www.askmedi.com). There is a charge for this service of about $15.

Yet one more way to check up on your candidates is through your state medical board. In most states, the names of disciplined doctors appear on the state's webpages. You can access all the states' sites by going to www.citizen.org/hrg/publications/1506.htm.

Questions for Yourself

While you're asking the doctor questions, you should also be considering some other issues that can be critical when it comes to making your decision. Some of the following questions may be much more important to you than others. Make a list of these questions as well, and note how you answer them.

- Do the doctor's actions and words make you feel comfortable?
- Does the doctor answer your questions politely and patiently, or is he or she condescending?
- If you are considering other cosmetic procedures in addition to Botox, is the doctor qualified to do these procedures?
- Does the doctor seem to be genuinely interested in your ideas and concerns?

- Do you feel as if you have the doctor's full attention during your interview? Do you feel rushed or pressured to hurry through your questions?
- Do you feel pressured to make a quick decision about treatment?
- Are the office hours convenient for you?
- Is the office conveniently located?
- Is the office staff polite and helpful?
- Are the waiting room and treatment rooms comfortable?
- How can the doctor be reached in case of emergency? At night and on weekends?

THE COST OF COSMETIC PROCEDURES

Beauty can be an expensive proposition. That's demonstrated by the fact that Americans spend billions of dollars a year on thousands of different beauty products and dozens of different procedures. All of those options have a cost, and many of them are a bit hard on the wallet, especially since cosmetic procedures are not covered by insurance. But when it comes to putting their best face forward, many women and men are willing to pay the price.

What is that price? We've gathered together the average price ranges for the cosmetic procedures discussed in this book. Naturally, prices vary depending on the part of the country in which you live and what the market will bear in your area.

The Price of Botox
The average price of Botox treatments for facial wrinkles is $200 to $600 per area treated (forehead wrinkles, frown

lines, and crow's-feet each being one area) or $10 to $20 per unit of Botox. When it comes to determining how doctors charge for those injections, some charge by the area treated, others by the units of Botox used. New York dermatologist John F. Romano, who is also assistant professor of dermatology at New York Weill Cornell Medical Center, says that pricing is an issue that's still developing. He notes that it's difficult to determine what an average amount of Botox is for a given area. "For example, I had a doctor in my office practice on me and I practiced on him. I had no results from what was considered to be an average amount, but he did well."

If someone has large frown muscles above their eyes, he says, they may require more Botox to get the desired result. "Men may have thicker muscles and may require twice as much of the drug as a woman," he says. "Since the drug is expensive, it probably makes sense to charge by the unit, because there's no one set amount that will be injected for everyone."

Palm Springs dermatologist Ronald Fragen agrees that unit pricing is better than paying by the area. "If the patient feels she didn't get enough, she can come back and get a bit more and only pay for what she gets," he says.

How can you know how much Botox you are getting? Leslie Baumann, MD, explains what consumers should consider when looking at price. "Patients should beware of any physician who prices Botox treatments too low," she warns. "They are obviously trying to build their practice, which means they probably have less experience using it. They often dilute the Botox with more saline than the physicians who have a lot of experience with the drug. This helps them keep their cost down."

She explains that most physicians dilute the Botox (which is delivered to doctors in an undiluted form) with 2.5 cc of saline per unit of Botox, which was the amount used during the FDA trials. Some doctors, however, dilute the drug with up to 10 cc, which means patients get a much less potent treatment that will not last as long. This greater dilution, however, allows doctors to get many more treatments out of each vial and thus make a bigger profit. "You may seem like you're getting a deal, but you will need to be injected much more often," she says.

Currently, doctors pay about $390 for each 100-unit vial of Botox. Each treatment site on the face typically requires 20 to 35 units, so doctors can potentially treat three to five areas with each vial.

During your consultation, the doctor should evaluate your face and try to determine how thick the muscles are and whether you may need more or less of the drug. Ask your doctor how much Botox he or she will be using for your treatment. The price should fall into a range of $10 to $20 per unit administered.

Finding the right doctor for your Botox injections, and for any possible additional cosmetic procedures, is important. This individual will literally have your face in his or her hands. Don't trust that face to just anyone!

You're finally ready to take the next big step: the consultation and then the treatment itself. In the next chapter, we discuss how a consultation might be done, and then we take you through the treatment process.

QUESTIONS AND ANSWERS

My general practitioner learned how to give Botox injections and has treated dozens of patients without any problem.

Now he's advertising Botox treatments for wrinkles. Why shouldn't I go to him for my injections?

Not all dermatologists, cosmetic surgeons, ophthalmologists, and ear-nose-throat surgeons agree that they are the only ones qualified to administer this drug. Some do argue that as long as doctors—be they general practitioners, internists, or neurologists—completely understand the risks involved, learn how to inject it and where, and develop an appreciation for the nuances of treatment, they should be allowed to give the injections. They insist that with practice, any doctor can become proficient in the techniques.

But before you go to your general practitioner for Botox, consider this. Who is best qualified to do the procedure you want? Would you go to your general practitioner to have a face-lift or a collagen injection to eliminate your laugh lines? Not likely. So why not go to someone who can guide and counsel you on what's best for your face? Why not establish a relationship with a doctor whom you may call upon later to do other cosmetic procedures?

In the end, the choice is up to you. We recommend, however, that you consider all the factors before making your decision.

There are skin clinics and spas offering Botox injections in my city. Are they safe places to have the procedure done?

If the individuals giving the injections are fully qualified physicians and you can interview them and have a consultation before your treatment, then there should be no reason why you shouldn't patronize these facilities. However, we strongly recommend you avoid any place in which nurse practitioners, physicians' assistants, or other individuals are the ones giving the injections, especially without a doctor's supervision.

Gary Monheit, MD, associate professor in the department of dermatology at the University of Alabama Medical Center in Birmingham, stresses the importance of choosing a qualified physician. "I understand that there are some nurses and cosmetologists giving Botox injections, some under the supervision of physicians and some without," he says. "I don't think it's good medicine for nonphysicians to administer Botox, especially when done without a physician present. This is a potentially toxic chemical that needs physician administration and supervision."

I want to get Botox, but I have a real fear of needles. I feel foolish telling the doctor this. What should I do?

The fear of needles is very common, and you shouldn't feel embarrassed. *Do* tell your doctor about your fears. She or he has heard it before, and there are ways to make the experience painless, both physically and emotionally. The time to reveal your concerns is during the interview or consultation; that is, preferably before the day you're getting treatment. That way, the doctor can explain the options you have to help you through the experience. See chapter 7 for information on what many doctors do to help make the injections a breeze.

I went to a doctor recommended by my best friend, who was thrilled with her treatments. But the doctor made me uncomfortable; I didn't feel like she was listening to my concerns. Am I being overly sensitive?

No. Different strokes for different folks. You can't expect to like everyone your best friend likes. If you were not comfortable with the doctor, then find another one. It's your face, and you need to feel good about who will be handling it. And if your best friend is *really* a friend, she won't care that you don't share her views on her doctor.

I went for a Botox consultation to talk about removing the wrinkles around my mouth, and the doctor told me she didn't recommend Botox for that area. She then recommended several other procedures instead. I got angry and didn't go back. Shouldn't I get what I want?

Although it's true that Botox can be used to help soften lines and wrinkles around the mouth, it is not as effective in these areas. Some doctors don't give injections in the mouth region for that reason. It is common for people to have other cosmetic procedures, such as dermabrasion, chemical peels, and injections of fillers such as collagen and fat, either along with Botox or as the only treatment, in this area of the face in order to get the best results.

Since you're not happy with the advice from the first doctor, you should probably get a second and even a third opinion and then weigh the information you get from all the doctors. Although Botox can be a great way to eliminate some wrinkles, it isn't always the answer.

My husband and I just moved across country. I'd like to get Botox treatments, but I don't know any of the doctors or hospitals in our new location, and I don't have friends to ask. How can I find a competent doctor?

You can contact any one or more of the following organizations and ask for a list of qualified individuals in your area: American Board of Plastic Surgery, 215-587-9322; American

Board of Dermatology, 313-874-1088; American Board of Ophthalmology, 610-664-1175; and American Board of Otolaryngology, 713-528-6200. Being board-certified in one of these specialties does not mean a doctor has the skill to administer Botox, however. You can consult the website www.botox.com, where you can see a list of doctors who have been trained in the administration of Botox. You can also check a doctor's certification status at the American Medical Association's Physician Select, which is an online service. It can be found at www.ama-assn.org/aps/amahg.htm. One more place to check is your state's medical board. Information for all states can be found at www.citizen.org/hrg/publications/1506.htm.

7

WHAT TO EXPECT AT
THE DOCTOR'S OFFICE

YOU'VE MADE THE DECISION to get Botox injections. You've done your homework. You believe you have realistic expectations about what the injections can and can't do for you. You've found a doctor who makes you feel comfortable and who is knowledgeable and experienced in giving Botox injections and in any other procedure you may be considering.

In this chapter, we take you through a typical experience with Botox. We begin with the consultation and then lead you through the preinjection preparations, the injections themselves, post-procedure guidelines, and your return visits. Even though your experience will not be exactly the same as the one we describe, it should be similar, as it portrays a professional, caring approach.

THE PRETREATMENT CONSULTATION

Once you've chosen the doctor who will do your procedure, it's time for your pretreatment consultation. Whether this is your first or second visit with the doctor, this is the time to ask any questions you have about Botox and the procedure itself, and also to make sure you and the doctor are on the same page when it comes to how you can rejuvenate and enhance your skin. You will be establishing a relationship that will hopefully last for many years, and one that has the potential to help change how you look and feel for the rest of your life.

IMPORTANCE OF A CONSULTATION

The value of seeking your cosmetic rejuvenation care from a qualified professional who conducts a thorough pretreatment consultation can't be emphasized enough. With the increasing number of cosmetic procedures and techniques available, you should consult with someone who can explain all your options. If you want to get the best results possible, it pays for you to take the time for a consultation.

Roberta D. Sengelmann, MD, assistant professor of dermatology and otolaryngology and director of the Center for Dermatologic and Cosmetic Surgery at Washington University School of Medicine in St. Louis, has been administering Botox for cosmetic enhancement for almost six years. She believes that a comprehensive consultation is essential.

"I want to understand what my patients are looking for," she says. "Generally, I do a consultation a few days to a few weeks before the procedure, and only rarely do we do it on the same day." The first priority for Dr. Sengelmann is for patients to talk about their concerns. "I'd say that at least 30 percent of the people who come to me saying they want a Botox consult don't need Botox as much as they need something else," she says. "They may think they need Botox, but they actually need a brow-lift or collagen injections, or another procedure to achieve their goals. Some patients think Botox is the answer to all of their woes, but, in fact, it's not. It's just one drug in a large armamentarium that can help us improve facial symmetry and appearance."

The Science of Botox

Dr. Sengelmann firmly believes that facial aesthetic enhancement is a whole science in and of itself, starting with skin care and sun protection and going on to tissue augmentation (such as collagen or fat injections), laser treatments, Botox, and even cosmetic dentistry.

"I look at the bone, muscle, soft tissues, and skin—there are at least four components that have to do with aging," she explains. "When I meet with a patient, I look at all four. Then I evaluate what I see and decide what they need. Many patients don't know exactly what they need because that requires a level of sophistication they wouldn't have. And why should they? It takes a lot of training to understand all the nuances of cosmetic enhancement." And part of the job of a good doctor well versed in cosmetic procedures is to help you realize your skin's potential.

Health and Medical Issues

Make sure you address all health and medical issues during your consultation. There are some conditions that may either exclude you from getting Botox injections and other treatments entirely or may simply require you to wait until your situation changes.

For example, if you have a disease that causes muscle deterioration, muscle weakness, and/or inflammation, such as myasthenia gravis, polymyositis, multiple sclerosis, or Lou Gehrig's disease, or an allergy to human albumin, which is an additive ingredient in Botox injections, then you should not get the drug. If you have Bell's palsy (paralysis of the face caused by a lesion of the facial nerve) or have had any type of facial paralysis, say, from a stroke, you should not get Botox. You can discuss other cosmetic options with the doctor.

When it comes to pregnancy and breast-feeding, there have not been any studies to identify whether the toxin passes through the placenta or is present in breast milk. However, most doctors recommend that their pregnant or breast-feeding patients wait until their situation changes before they get Botox, or perhaps choose another cosmetic procedure.

Generally, conditions such as heart disease, high blood pressure, diabetes, or cancer are not reasons to forgo Botox injections. However, if you have any medical concerns, make sure to mention them to your doctor.

You also need to discuss which over-the-counter or prescription medications and herbs you should avoid before the procedure. Those that cause thinning of the blood should be avoided for one to two weeks before treatment, if possible. They include:

- Aspirin and other nonsteroidal anti-inflammatory drugs (e.g., ibuprofen, indomethacin, naproxen)
- Warfarin (Coumadin)
- Vitamin E
- Ginkgo biloba
- St. John's wort
- Feverfew

- Garlic tablets
- Herbal supplements (discuss with your doctor)

The risk of getting a bruise is increased if a patient continues to use these substances. Even with their use, the risk is small, but Dr. Sengelmann likes to let patients know in advance that bruising is a possibility. "They won't be too pleased if you didn't tell them ahead of time," she says, "especially if they are in the public eye or have a big event to attend soon after their treatment."

Warning: Drugs That Don't Mix with Botox

Although there do not appear to be any significant interactions between Botox and most other drugs, there are a few medications that can cause severe muscle weakness if they are being taken by individuals who get Botox. The manufacturer of Botox therefore recommends that people who are taking the following drugs not get Botox injections:

- Calcium channel blockers (e.g., diltiazem, nifedipine, verapamil)
- Aminoglycosides (e.g., amikacin, gentamicin, tobramycin)
- Quinine
- Penicillamine

If you are taking one of these medications, you and your doctor can discuss other cosmetic procedure options.

The Key to Success

"Basically, a successful consultation comes down to good communication," says Dr. Sengelmann. "I tell my patients to come in so we can talk. I want them to tell me what they don't like about their face, I tell them what I think, and then I explain other procedures that I don't think will be helpful, but about which I think they should be aware because they'll probably read about them in a magazine and they should be informed." This is also the time to get estimates for any procedures and to talk about payment options (see pricing information in chapter 6).

After the consultation, it's all up to you. Weigh everything you've discussed with your doctor and how you feel about it. Do you feel comfortable with the doctor and his or her staff? Do you believe the results that have been explained to you are what you want? Do you understand how the procedure will be performed? Do you understand the costs? Once you feel confident you have all the answers you need and you feel good about them, you're ready to make the appointment for your treatment.

SETTING THE SCENE FOR TREATMENT

We realize that every doctor approaches and handles his or her patients differently, so the scenario we give here will probably not be exactly like the one you experience. We hope that it will be similar, however, because it represents an approach offered by the many professionals who provide cosmetic enhancement. Also, the description we give here assumes the injections are being given on the upper third of the face for elimination of forehead lines, frown lines, and crow's-feet. Treatment procedures for other areas of the face or to the neck may differ.

Do You Need an Anesthetic?

Beauty shouldn't have to hurt. That's the consensus of doctors and patients alike when it comes to Botox injections. Everyone has his or her own pain threshold, so the use of a topical anesthetic before getting Botox injections is a personal choice. However, all doctors *should* offer you that choice, and in fact most do. Similarly, many patients do take their doctors up on the offer.

During her consultation, Teresa, a forty-nine-year-old sales executive, sheepishly told her doctor that she was terrified of needles. "I've had this fear my entire life," she says. "But I don't want it to stop my getting the injections. I wanted my doctor to reassure me that I wouldn't feel the needles."

Teresa's doctor recommended that she apply a topical anesthetic to her forehead about 30 minutes before she was scheduled for her treatment. Although there is an over-the-counter product available, Teresa asked for a prescription, and her doctor gave her one for a lidocaine and prilocaine combination (brand name EMLA, or Eutetic Mixture of Local Anesthetics). Use of this anesthetic, along with the application of ice to her forehead at the time of injection, reassured Teresa that she would barely feel the needle sticks.

It's your choice whether you want to use a topical anesthetic. Ask your doctor about it during your consultation. In addition to EMLA, other lidocaine and prilocaine combination products are Betacaine (which is only available through the manufacturer), and Ela-Max (which is an over-the-counter product). Consult with your doctor for more information and always be sure to mention any allergies you may have to lidocaine and other -caine derivative drugs.

Side Effects of Topical Anesthetics

These topical anesthetics are not without side effects and some minor inconvenience. EMLA can cause paleness at the application site (occurs in 37 percent of people), redness (30 percent), swelling (6 percent), and itching (2 percent). (Severe allergic reactions occur in less than 1 percent, with rare reports of death as a result.) These reactions generally disappear in about one to two hours. EMLA also requires that you place a piece of plastic wrap (the kind you use to wrap leftovers) over the treated spot until you are ready for the injections. ELA-Max and Betacaine do not require you to use plastic wrap, but they can cause redness that may linger for several hours.

Menstruation and Pain

Teresa is in menopause, or else her doctor might also have suggested that she not get her injections during menstruation. Many women are more sensitive to pain during their period. If you are concerned about pain and needles, you may feel more comfortable if you wait until your menstrual cycle is over to receive your Botox treatment.

GETTING READY FOR THE INJECTIONS

Before you sit down for your injections, the doctor will quickly review the procedure with you to make sure you understand what is going to take place. This is the time to ask any last-minute questions. Then you'll be asked to sign a consent form and to pose for your "before" photo. Then you're ready for your injections.

The procedure is done while you are sitting upright or slightly leaning back in a chair. After your face is cleaned with alcohol, you'll be asked to frown, squint, or otherwise contract your facial muscles so the doctor can see the areas to be treated. She or he will mark the areas with a surgical pen, and then an ice pack may be applied to the area as an anesthetic. The ice also helps minimize any bleeding. If you've already applied a topical painkiller, the ice provides an additional numbing effect.

THE INJECTIONS

You may be given a small rubber ball or other soft object to squeeze while the doctor makes the injections. Some patients choose to hold the hand of the doctor's assistant, while others are fine without any support. The doctor will then take a 30- or 32-gauge needle (both are very tiny, and most patients can't tell the difference between the two) and make a series of injections into the areas she has marked. Treatment can take from 5 to 15 minutes, depending on the number of injections needed. The average amount of Botox injected is 15 to 35 units per area (that is, 15 to 35 units for complete treatment of forehead lines, etc.).

How many needle sticks can you expect? Generally, here's how the doctor will treat your face and the muscles she will inject (see the box and the illustration, "Name That Muscle"):

- Forehead lines: four to eight injections across the middle of the forehead (into the frontalis muscle) between your scalp and your eyebrows, and then several injections on each side.

- Frown lines: five to seven injections into the glabellar frown complex between the brows. This includes four muscles: corrugator supercilii, procerus, orbicularis oculi, and depressor supercilii.

- Crow's-feet: two to four injections into the orbicularis oculi muscle at the corner of each eye and wrapping down onto the cheek

- Other areas: areas above and around the mouth, the neck, the bunny lines of the nose, and the lower eyelid typically require a combination of procedures, and the number of needle sticks varies.

Again, depending on the areas treated, the doctor will gently massage each injection site to help disperse the drug. The area directly over the brow is not massaged because doing so may cause the drug to drift down into an adjacent muscle and cause a drooping eyelid. (See chapter 8 for information on drooping eyelids.)

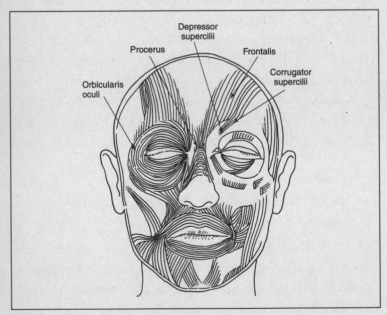

Name That Muscle

Name That Muscle

Your facial expressions are the result of more than 50 muscles, different ones of which work together to produce the smiles, frowns, scowls, and other looks you present to the world. Here's a brief description of the muscles that are most often treated with Botox and what they do. See the illustration for the location of these muscles.

- **Frontalis:** responsible for the horizontal lines in your forehead. It is also the muscle that you contract when you want to raise your eyebrows.

- **Procurus:** responsible for the horizontal line over the top of the nose and partly responsible for the vertical frown lines between your eyebrows.

- **Depressor supercilii:** causes your eyebrows to pull down.

- **Corrugator supercilii:** causes your eyebrows to partly pull down; responsible for the vertical furrows between your brows.

- **Orbicularis oculi:** closes the eye; responsible for the formation of crow's-feet.

A FEW POST-PROCEDURE TIPS

You're all done! Now you can relax, unclench your fists, and talk to your doctor about how you feel it went. Remember that although the procedure is over, it usually takes three to seven days to see the full results of your treatment. That's how long it takes for the toxin to have its full effect on the nerves/muscles that were treated. Before you leave the office, you'll be given an appointment for a follow-up visit in two to three weeks, and some post-procedure instructions. They are simple:

- Use your muscles. You should use your facial muscles to maximum contraction for about 20 minutes after the procedure. That means if you had injections to eliminate your frown lines, you should frown; if you went in to get rid of crow's-feet, you should squint; and if you were treated for worry lines, you should raise your eyebrows and look surprised. If you had more than one of these areas treated, you will be combining your expressions and making some pretty funny faces on your way home. But there is a scientific reason for these expressions says Dr. Sengelmann. "The theory is that Botox is taken up by the active muscles, which is where we want it," she explains. Your 20 minutes of intense muscle activity will help ensure Botox works to your best advantage in tackling those annoying wrinkles.

- Stay upright. This is a safety precaution to prevent any possible drifting of the toxin into other muscles of the face. Generally, don't lie flat for three to four hours after the procedure.

- Don't overdo it. Avoid bending over and vigorous exercise, including dancing, for up to four hours after the injections. Again, this is a safety precaution to avoid diffusion of the Botox.

- Ice if needed. A small percentage of people experience bruising at the injection sites. You can apply ice (a frozen bag of peas will do just fine) to relieve this problem. A study at the University of Miami found that applying vitamin K cream twice a day to the injection sites also speeds up resolution of bruising. The homeopathic compound arnica (cream) also may help.

- Enjoy it! Frieda had her first Botox treatment on a Friday afternoon after work, before a long Memorial Day weekend. When she returned to work the following Tuesday, the drug had already taken effect. "Several of my coworkers commented on how rested I looked," she said. "They had no idea I had had the injections. I felt great, and I knew I looked great."

Follow-Up Visit

If this is your first Botox treatment, you need to schedule a follow-up visit for two to three weeks after your injections. This is an opportunity not only for the doctor to get those essential "after treatment" photos, but also to discuss any questions you may have. The doctor can evaluate the treated areas and, if necessary, do a touch-up injection. The need for touch-up occurs in about 2 percent of cases. Why?

Say you had your forehead lines treated. The frontalis muscle on one side of your forehead may be stronger than the frontalis muscle on the other side. If the doctor used the same dosage of Botox throughout, the stronger muscle may still be working more than the other, which may make your forehead look asymmetrical. Or you may have especially strong forehead muscles and require a higher dose overall. In either case, a quick injection can take care of the situation.

The follow-up visit is also an opportunity for you to reflect on your new look. Now that you know what's possible with Botox, you might think about whether you want to keep having the injections and whether you want to undergo any other cosmetic enhancements sometime in the future. Some patients decide that next time they would like to treat a different area or inject a little bit more of the drug. Use this visit to evaluate the results of your treatment with your doctor.

YOUR NEXT TREATMENT

Usually about four to five months after your treatment, you'll begin to notice lines and wrinkles returning to the treated area. Some people don't see a change in the treated area for six months. When should you make an appointment for your next treatment: when the wrinkles first start to return, or when they've already come back?

"I generally tell people to come back when they first start noticing that the effect is wearing off," says Ronald Fragen, MD. "That's because if you inject a muscle that is weakened, the Botox will work better and last longer. If you wait for the muscle to get back all its strength, then you're injecting a stronger muscle, and it takes more units of Botox to do that. It's like starting all over again."

Botox does seem to have a cumulative effect. That does *not* mean the toxin builds up to dangerous levels in your body. What it means is this: people who have received several treatments have had their muscles weakened continuously for twelve months or longer, and they may find that the interval between injections is six to eight months rather than four to six, because the muscles are accustomed to being in a weakened state. But, doctors say, the intervals vary from person to person and cannot be predicted with certainty. Dr. Sengelmann, who has some patients she's been treating with Botox for six years, says that most of them return at five- to six-month intervals.

QUESTIONS AND ANSWERS

I got my first Botox treatment for forehead wrinkles six days ago and I'm not seeing results yet. My sister had a Botox treatment on a Monday, and she had results by Wednesday.

Typically, it takes one to five days for the muscles to relax enough for you to see results. However, this is the average. Some people don't see results for a week or more. By your follow-up visit, which is usually two to three weeks after your injections, you should be seeing the full benefits of your treatment.

It's also possible that you may need a little bit more Botox injected into the area that was treated. Your doctor can take care of that during your follow-up visit. About 2 percent of people need a "touch-up" treatment to relax a muscle that is perhaps a bit stronger than the others.

I take ibuprofen for arthritis pain. Do I have to stop taking it a week or two before my Botox injections? I really don't want to.

Before undergoing Botox injections, doctors typically suggest that patients stop taking any type of drug, vitamin, or herb that can cause blood-thinning. This is merely a precaution against the possibility of slight bruising where the injections are given. Naturally, your doctor doesn't want you to suffer, so you don't need to stop any medication you are taking for pain. You just deserve to know that minor bruising *may* occur if you are taking a substance that can thin your blood. After your Botox injections, you can use an ice pack to reduce bruising and a little bit of makeup to cover any discoloration at the injection sites. Any bruising that may occur normally disappears within several days.

A friend told me that I can get Botox injections for the creases in my neck. How safe is this procedure?

Injecting Botox into the neck to eliminate wrinkles requires a doctor who is well trained and cautious. Dr. Sengelmann warns that if the injections are not given properly, you can develop complications, including difficulty swallowing. Because the area being treated is larger, the number of units injected is greater, but it should never be more than 200, says Dr. Sengelmann.

Leslie Baumann, MD, director of cosmetic dermatology at the University of Miami Medical School, says that Botox injections for neck wrinkles provide minimal results, and that patients experience bruising and risk a loss of neck muscle strength.

Can I put on makeup immediately after getting Botox injections?

Yes, there's no reason why you can't apply your makeup immediately afterward. Botox injections do not affect the skin in any way, nor do they leave any tell-tale signs, except for some minor bruising in some cases, which can be covered up with makeup.

Why can't I lie down while getting my Botox injections? I think I'd feel more comfortable that way.

The reason you will be sitting upright (or leaning back slightly) is to prevent the possibility of the drug drifting beyond the area that is being treated and causing a complication, such as a drooping eyelid.

If you have any concerns about your comfort during the procedure, make sure you talk about them with your doctor at your consultation. If you are concerned about possible pain, your doctor can suggest a topical anesthetic for you to apply before you come to the office. Perhaps you can hold the hand of the doctor's assistant during the injections. Whatever your concerns are, your doctor will make every attempt to make your experience a comfortable and rewarding one.

Will I need to have someone drive me home after my Botox treatment?

One of the beauties of Botox treatments is that there is no downtime associated with the procedure. That's why they call it a "lunch-time" cosmetic procedure. You should be perfectly able to drive yourself home after your injections.

My doctor said I may want to schedule my Botox injections when I'm not having my period. Why did she make that suggestion?

Your doctor was very thoughtful to make that suggestion. Some women are more susceptible to pain during menstruation. If you are sensitive to needles, you may feel more comfortable if you have the injections when you're not menstruating.

8

SATISFACTION GUARANTEED? WHAT YOU NEED TO KNOW ABOUT SIDE EFFECTS AND COMPLICATIONS

WHEN YOU TALK TO DOCTORS who are experienced at giving Botox injections for cosmetic enhancement, their comments begin to sound like a broken record: "I haven't had a problem in years." "My patients love it. I never have a problem." "Side effects are rare. If you know what you're doing, there's no problem."

These are reassuring words. Indeed, reported side effects from cosmetic use of Botox have been few. Most patients and their doctors are happy with the drug. But nothing is perfect. Side effects, even though they may be mild and temporary, do occur.

One concern that has arisen in the minds of many doctors is that while adverse reactions have been relatively scarce in the past, they may increase as the number of Botox treatments surges. At the same time, more side effects and complications may result from the injections being administered by individuals, physicians and nonphysicians, who are not familiar with the muscles in the face or with cosmetic procedures.

If, however, you do your homework and find a competent, experienced practitioner who can address all your questions, concerns, and cosmetic rejuvenation needs, then your chance of experiencing any significant problems is extremely low. The guidelines discussed in chapter 6 can help you find such a practitioner.

That being said, you should be aware of the possible side effects related to cosmetic use of Botox. In this chapter, we discuss those adverse effects, how and why they may occur, and what you can do about them. We also look at another "side effect" of Botox: the social/cultural implications of its use.

SIDE EFFECTS AND COMPLICATIONS

The majority of physicians seem to agree that when Botox is administered by a competent, cautious doctor, the side effects are very mild and minor, and that anything serious is rare. With that in mind, let's look at some of the complications that are associated with the cosmetic use of Botox.

Before any drug is introduced to the general public, it must first undergo several phases of testing. In clinical trials that tested the cosmetic use of Botox against a placebo, the manufacturer notes that the most frequently reported side effects were headache, respiratory infection, drooping eyelid, nausea, and flu symptoms. Side effects that occurred even less frequently included face pain, redness at the injection site, and muscle weakness.

When the incidence and frequency of side effects associated with Botox were compared with placebo, says Roberta

D. Sengelmann, MD, assistant professor of dermatology and otolaryngology and director of the Center for Dermatologic & Cosmetic Surgery at Washington University School of Medicine in St. Louis, there was very little difference between the two. She believes this is due to the fact that the drug stays where it's injected and acts locally, and that very little of the drug is absorbed by the body. When the rate of side effects during treatment with a drug is the same as or less than that in the placebo group, odds are that the reactions are due to extraneous causes and are not attributable to the drug at all.

The one exception was drooping eyelid. It occurred in 3 percent of those who received Botox and in 0 percent of those who got a placebo, and thus can be directly attributed to the Botox treatment. The reason for this is diffusion of Botox into an adjacent muscle that lifts the eyelid and lets it relax, causing a temporarily drooping eyelid.

Drooping Eyelid and Lip Asymmetry

When treating the glabellar frown complex in the forehead, an injection that is placed too close to the eyelid can drift down and weaken the levator muscle. When this muscle is weakened, the eyelid droops, and it becomes difficult to lift your eyelid. Generally, this complication affects 1 percent of patients and causes a 1- to 3-mm lid droop, which resolves spontaneously in three weeks. In addition, there are drugs that can counteract this complication if it occurs, including iopidine and neosynephrine.

Injections of Botox around the mouth, which are typically done along with wrinkle fillers or laser resurfacing, must be done with great care. The amount of the drug given around the mouth is typically less than is injected in the upper part of the face, and administering too much can cause excessive weakening of the muscles, causing lip asymmetry. It may be temporarily challenging to manipulate large bites of food and to swish without accidentally spitting.

Headache

If you get a headache after receiving Botox, you can expect it to be mild and to last for no more than 12 hours after treatment. But in a few rare cases, the pain can be longer lasting and severe. That was the finding of researchers who published their findings in the *Journal of the American Academy of Dermatology* in January 2002. In a group of 320 people who received Botox for cosmetic enhancement, four developed severe, constant headaches that lasted for two to four weeks. Attempts to treat the pain with typical headache medication didn't bring much relief. Eventually, the pain subsided in all four patients.

Bruising

Mild bruising at the injection sites may occur. It is more likely to occur if you taking any type of medication, vitamin, or herb that can thin the blood (e.g., feverfew, St. John's wort, ginkgo biloba, aspirin, warfarin). Because the injections are made into very thin tissues, says Ronald Fragen, MD, of Fragen Cosmetic Surgery Center in Palm Springs, California, it's possible to hit a capillary and cause a bruise.

You can help get rid of any unsightly discoloration by placing an ice pack on the sites. Makeup can be applied immediately after treatment as well. One study also reports that rubbing vitamin K cream on bruises will speed up their disappearance. Any bruising that occurs usually disappears in several days.

Other Side Effects

The rates of respiratory infections, nausea, and flu symptoms in both the patients who received Botox and those who got placebo in the FDA trial were so similar and low that they appear to be insignificant. Other complications, though rare, that have been associated with Botox injections include:

- Worsening of eyebrow droop, if it was significant before your Botox injections (occurs in less than 1 percent of patients).
- Double vision or crossed eyes when injections are given near the eyes (only a few cases reported).
- Injections near the mouth may limit your ability to whistle or use a straw.
- Injections given in the neck to eliminate wrinkles in that area can result in a loss of neck muscle strength and difficulty swallowing (both of which resolve in several weeks).
- Decreased tear production.

All of these adverse reactions are temporary, lasting from a few weeks to a few months at most.

WHEN BOTOX DOESN'T WORK

In a very small percentage of people, Botox reportedly doesn't work at all. Joanne, a fifty-six-year-old museum curator, was excited about getting her first Botox injections for

crow's-feet and frown lines. She sailed through the procedure, went home full of anticipation, and a month later was
still waiting for results.

"I was so disappointed," she said. "My doctor had mentioned that a very small percentage of people don't respond,
but I just thought, well, he has to say that to everybody, but I
wouldn't be one of those people. But I was."

Joanne did go back and get a stronger dose a second time
to see if she would respond, but when she got minimal results, she decided not to pursue it any longer.

Why Some People Don't Respond

How come some people don't respond to the injections?
Dr. Fragen believes it has to do with an individual's ability to
break down the medicine. Unfortunately, he says, there's no
way to know beforehand how a person will respond. "I always tell people before the procedure that they may need
more. I find in people who are initially more resistant that if I
give them a higher concentration of drug in the injection, it
seems to last longer and they respond better. But for some
people, it just doesn't work well."

He notes that some people normally have stronger forehead
or frown muscles, which can make them more resistant to the
drug. If you have heavy muscles in your forehead, which is
more common among men but is also found in women, you
may need a few more units to adequately relax the muscles.

Every doctor's experience with Botox is not exactly the
same. "I've used Botox for nearly six years, and I've never
had someone not respond," says Dr. Sengelmann. "People
who don't respond may not have gotten enough of the drug.
If you get enough Botox into the muscle, you'll get a re-

sponse. If you don't get the kind of results you want, it's important to communicate that to your doctor."

Dr. Sengelmann recommends that patients always wait at least two weeks after treatment to allow time for the Botox to work. If you still don't see results, then it's time to talk to your doctor. "When you see your doctor, ask how many units you were given and how your outcome can be improved," she says.

Immunity to Botox

Another rare occurrence is immunity. According to Gary D. Monheit, MD, associate professor in the department of dermatology at the University of Alabama Medical Center in Birmingham, there is a "potential theoretical problem of the building up of antibodies against the botulinum molecule, which would make the drug less effective with repeated use." This immunity to the toxin has been seen in people who are receiving Botox for medical conditions, because the number of units they receive at each treatment is often much greater (perhaps eight times higher or more) than those used for cosmetic purposes. As far as Dr. Monheit knows, immunity has never occurred in association with cosmetic use of Botox.

In 1997, a new, reformulated batch of the drug was introduced. Prior to that time, the batch from which all the injections were created had a higher protein content than the newer mixture. Experts theorize that the decrease in protein has reduced the risk of antibody formation and thus the potential development of resistance to the drug.

What You Can Do

Nothing speaks louder than results. If two weeks after your treatment you have a poor response to the injections, make sure you keep your follow-up appointment and talk to your doctor about what can be done to resolve the situation. Lack of an adequate response is virtually always due to inadequate dosing, which varies from one person to another. As we've said, immunity has never been substantiated with cosmetic use of Botox. Either of these concerns or others must be discussed with your doctor.

For now, there's no way of knowing before treatment whether an individual will respond or whether immunity will develop. However, the percentage of people who experience either immunity or a poor response is very low, especially among those who get Botox to treat wrinkles.

If you are among the rare few who don't respond well to Botox, take heart. You can try another cosmetic procedure, such as dermabrasion, chemical peels, or injection with a wrinkle filler, such as collagen, to get the look you want. We talk about these and other ways to treat wrinkles in chapter 9.

BOTOX: SOCIAL IMPLICATIONS

When people talk about getting Botox injections to improve their appearance and to look younger, they almost never bring up the possible negative side of this trend. Is there a downside to wanting to look younger and wrinkle-free?

Gerontologist Robert N. Butler, founder of the International Longevity Center in New York City and Pulitzer Prize–winning author of *Why Survive? Being Old in America,* is concerned about the impact of aging and longevity on society and believes we need to examine our obsession with looking young.

"If you have a Botox forehead, who's going to know if

you're frowning or what your emotional state is?" he says. He believes the use of Botox for cosmetic purposes "really depletes emotionality as well as reflects the concern that seems to be so common in our country, of wishing to be youthful."

Part of that concern comes from our growing tendency to label situations in our lives or even stages of life as a disease—something that has to be fixed, even though it's a natural part of the life cycle. We've seen that tendency with menopause, which certainly is a natural part of a woman's life, yet it is sometimes portrayed by the media and by some doctors as a disease. Now we are looking at aging, and wrinkles in particular, as a flaw of nature and as something that must be eliminated or "fixed." In other words, we are redefining aging as a disease.

"Some of it [our redefining of what a medical condition truly is] may be answerable in terms of cultural expectations, job needs, and social requirements," Dr. Butler says, "but nevertheless it needs to be discussed." But unfortunately, he says, it's a topic that is rarely talked about.

One forty-something woman has this perspective: "For each of us, it comes down to a matter of priorities, personal choice, and a lot of soul-searching. Personally, I will wear each and every one of my lines and wrinkles with pride. I earned them. I don't feel they diminish me. I refuse to succumb to what I think is a very self-centered and superficial way to value each other as human beings. We are not our wrinkles. Do I love my mother any less because she has wrinkles? No. Would I love her more if she suddenly didn't have them? No. But that's just my personal opinion. Everyone has the right to make their own choice when it comes to changing how they look."

QUESTIONS AND ANSWERS

The Food and Drug Administration (FDA) indicates that Botox is for people sixty-five years and younger. Does that mean it's not safe for people who are older?

Gary D. Monheit, MD, associate professor in the department of dermatology at the University of Alabama Medical Center, Birmingham, explains that the FDA placed this restriction on the drug because the criteria for the FDA testing were for people younger than sixty-five years old. That's why the FDA can only give its approval for people in the younger age group. However, many doctors have been and continue to give the injections to people who are older than sixty-five without complications. Doctors who are used to working with elderly skin recognize that extra care should be taken to avoid undue stress and pressure to the skin, because our skin gets thinner and more fragile with age.

I love my Botox treatments and plan to keep getting them for many years. But I'm a little worried about developing an immunity to it and then it won't be effective anymore. Could that really happen?

"There is a potential theoretical problem in which the body can build up antibodies against the botulinum molecule, which would make Botox less effective with repeated use," says Dr. Monheit. "This has been seen in neurologic conditions (e.g., crossed eyes, dystonias) where high doses are used, but we've never seen it in cosmetic uses in which smaller amounts are given at a time."

9

GOING BEYOND BOTOX: OTHER COSMETIC PROCEDURES

NOW IS AN EXCITING TIME to be considering skin rejuvenation, because there are so many options to choose from within your reach. Perhaps the changes you want to make cannot be achieved using Botox alone. In many cases, people decide to combine Botox injections with chemical peels, or collagen injections, or microdermabrasion, or they choose to have a Botox treatment now and a non-ablative laser treatment (that does not damage the outer layer of skin) later.

When you make your appointment for your consultation, it will help for you to have a general knowledge of the cosmetic procedures that are offered. That way, you'll feel better informed and more prepared to explore your options.

When you evaluated your face, you may have learned that some of the wrinkles and lines you want to eliminate are located in areas that are not best suited for Botox injections, typically those around the nose, mouth, and neck. Sometimes, Botox injections for forehead lines, frown lines, and crow's-feet may still need some additional touch-up from another procedure to achieve the look you want.

For example, if you have very deep forehead lines, your doctor may recommend using collagen or another injectable wrinkle filler along with Botox to eliminate them for you. Here's the reason: these deep wrinkles have two causes— muscle contraction and aging—and so are treated with two different approaches, one for each cause. The Botox relaxes the muscles while the filler takes care of the signs of the aging process; that is, the loss of collagen from the underlying layer of skin, or dermis.

The rest of this chapter focuses on those alternative cosmetic procedures and what you can expect from them. In particular, we discuss cosmetic procedures that, like Botox, involve no downtime, or just minimal time. Therefore, more invasive cosmetic procedures such as laser resurfacing, dermabrasion, and deep chemical peels are discussed only very briefly in this book. In many cases, the procedures discussed here can be used along with Botox injections to enhance your revitalized look.

With so many options from which to choose, making a decision can be confusing. That is why we have this caveat: regardless of the procedures you select, make sure you thoroughly investigate the qualifications of the doctor you choose for the procedure and the results he or she has had with it. The procedure or technique is only as good as the physician who performs it. We've already talked about how to find that medical professional in chapter 6.

Abbie's Story

Abbie had read a few articles about Botox and soon decided she had found the answer to her prayers. "I didn't want a face-lift," said the fifty-seven-year-old medical claims processor, "and I didn't want a chemical peel or laser resurfacing procedure that makes you look so bad you have to go into hiding for a week. Yet I didn't want to look at all those wrinkles anymore, especially those across my forehead and down the sides of my mouth." She contacted a cosmetic surgeon recommended by a friend and told him she wanted Botox for everything. Period.

During her consultation with the doctor, Abbie learned that while Botox would help with her forehead wrinkles, the best choice for her laugh lines would be collagen injections complemented with Botox injections.

"I didn't even know what collagen injections were before my doctor told me about them," she said. "I had read about Botox and just decided for myself that that's what I needed. I wish I had been a little more knowledgeable about my options before I went to my doctor. I just thought Botox would take care of everything. But after the doctor explained that I could get the results I wanted by combining the two procedures, I was ready to try it."

Abbie had both procedures done while her husband was away on a business trip. She waited anxiously to see his reaction. "When he came home, he said he thought he'd walked into the wrong house. He just loved the way I looked. Now he's talking about getting Botox for his frown lines."

WRINKLE FILLERS:
SOFT-TISSUE AUGMENTATION

Would you like to eliminate the lines that have taken up residence around your mouth? Do you love to smile but the thought of those etched-in laugh lines makes you frown? Are you tired of the lines that radiate from around your lips or the deep creases on either side of your mouth?

You've already learned that Botox can't take care of all the different types of wrinkles that can develop on the face. One approach that is especially helpful for those deeper lines that form around the mouth or drop down from the sides of your nose is the use of wrinkle fillers, also known as soft-tissue augmentation. Wrinkle fillers can be used alone or combined with other procedures, such as Botox injections, chemical peels, or laser treatments, to achieve the look you want. Benefits of getting wrinkle fillers are that the procedure can be done quickly (usually less than an hour) and in most cases you can return to work the same or next day.

Several wrinkle fillers are on the market, and more are expected to be approved by the Food and Drug Administration in the coming years. Today, among the most common ones in use are bovine collagen, autologous fat transfer (harvested from your own fat reserves), AlloDerm, Cymetra, SoftForm, and expanded polytetrafluoroethylene (ePTFE).

Bovine Collagen

Since bovine (cow) collagen injections were introduced in the early 1980s, tens of thousands of women and men have had the injections and found the filler to be a safe and effective way to soften lines and wrinkles, especially around the mouth. As we discussed in chapter 3, collagen is a protein that's found in the dermis, where it helps support the skin. As we age, that support begins to deteriorate, and then it's good-bye smooth, taut skin, hello wrinkles.

Bovine collagen is derived from cow skin that is purified, sterilized, and processed into a liquid. It is well tolerated by the majority of people, but about 3 to 5 percent of people are allergic to it, especially those who have an allergy to meat or dairy foods. To make sure you're not allergic to the injec-tions, your doctor will do a simple skin test on your arm and wait two weeks to see if there is a reaction (swelling, itching, redness). Most doctors conduct a second allergy test, just to make sure the results were correct. After the second skin test is done, you will need to wait another four weeks before going forward with the collagen injections. Although this delay may be annoying, it's worth the wait if it helps you avoid an allergic reaction. After two negative or nonreactive skin tests, the rate of allergy risk drops to about 1 percent.

Different Types of Bovine Collagen

Bovine collagen comes in three different viscosities (thick-ness or "gooeyness" of the collagen), and each one is de-signed to best treat a different type of line or wrinkle. The least viscous form is called Zyderm I and is best for mild fore-head wrinkles, frown lines, crow's-feet, and fine lines around the mouth and cheeks. Medium to deeper wrinkles are best treated with the next higher viscosity, a product called Zy-derm II, while deeper wrinkles, such as marionette lines and laugh (smile) lines, may respond best to the most viscous form, called Zyplast. Your doctor will decide which collagen will work best for you.

Like Botox injections, collagen injections are a "lunchtime" procedure that can be done in the doctor's office with no recovery time necessary. Also like Botox, however, you do need to return for repeat injections every few months, typically every three to six for collagen. The average cost of collagen injections is $350 to $550 per 1-cc syringe, which is adequate to do laugh lines.

Safety Precautions

To help ensure that your experience with bovine collagen is a safe one, there are some precautions and risks you and your doctor will need to discuss. We have made a list of some of the important ones. Take this list with you to be sure you have all your questions answered.

- In rare cases, people who have no history of a connective tissue disease have developed such a condition after receiving collagen injections. The two conditions that have been reported are polymyositis and dermatomyositis. So far, there is no definitive evidence that the injections have caused these disorders, but the possibility remains.

- Collagen injections should not be taken if you have had an allergic reaction to the skin test (given by your doctor before the decision to use collagen is made), to any other injectable collagen products, or to lidocaine. Also, you should not receive collagen injections if you are undergoing or have had desensitization injections to meat products (remember, bovine collagen is derived from cows).

- If you have a history of allergy to beef products, you should undergo more than one skin allergy test before deciding to get collagen injections.

- Approximately 1 to 2 percent of people develop an allergic reaction to collagen injections, even after they have tested negative on the skin tests. This response may include swelling, itching, firmness, and prolonged redness at the injection site(s). Rarely, cysts may develop and form a scar.

- Any injection has a risk of infection, although this is very rare. You may also experience mild bruising or discoloration at the injection site.

- If you have ever had facial herpes simplex at the injection site, an injection of collagen may stimulate a recurrence of the condition.

- Rarely, collagen may be mistakenly injected into a blood vessel, which can cause a blockage of the blood flow and a loss of blood circulation in the surrounding area. Accidental injection into a blood vessel may also cause temporary discoloration of the injection site or may lead to skin sloughing, resulting in the formation of a scab or scar.

- If you have a history of allergic reactions to other substances, or if you are receiving immunosuppressive therapy, such as prednisone or other steroids, injections of collagen should be given with caution.

- If you are experiencing some type of inflammatory skin condition, such as hives, rash, or a skin infection, you may be advised by your doctor to postpone your collagen injections until the condition clears.

- The safety of collagen injections during pregnancy has not been determined. If you are pregnant, you and your doctor need to discuss whether getting injections is right for you.

- Side effects from the injections are rare: fewer than two people per one thousand have reported symptoms such as dizziness, nausea, headache, rash, visual problems, breathing difficulties, and joint aches after treatment. These rates compare to those experienced by people who were given a placebo in studies, and hence may be due to chance alone.

Combining Botox and Collagen Injections

"Botox is great," says New York dermatologist Debra Jaliman, clinical instructor at Mount Sinai Medical School in New York, "but it doesn't do everything. People have to realize that, and then be willing to work with different techniques to achieve the most beautiful complexion."

Parda went to her dermatologist with the idea that Botox injections would solve all her wrinkle problems. She soon learned she was wrong.

"My doctor explained that while she recommended Botox for my frown lines and crow's-feet, she wanted me to consider other options for my marionette lines," said the thirty-nine-year-old advertising executive. "Of course, after she explained how injecting Botox into the muscles on the side of my mouth might leave me drooling for a few months, I was convinced that I needed to choose another procedure for those lines."

After learning about the advantages and disadvantages

of various injectables and implants, including bovine collagen, fat, and other fillers, Parda chose to have a small
amount of fat removed from her knee for the injections.
Five months after receiving her Botox injections and fat
injections, she was ready for her first repeat Botox treatment and was thrilled with the results of all her injections.

Fat Injections

Injecting fat, also known as autologous fat transfer, is a
procedure in which a small amount of fat is removed from a
part of your body, usually the buttocks, knees, thighs, or
stomach, using liposuction. The harvested fat is then used to
fill in deep wrinkles and other depressions of the skin associated with the aging process.

John F. Romano, MD, a New York dermatologist and assistant professor of dermatology at New York Weill Cornell
Medical Center, says, "It is a very reasonable thing to do in
some areas, especially when you need a lot of volume, such as
cheeks. It certainly lasts longer than collagen."

Using your own fat has several advantages. It's very natural looking, because it is, after all, you. Because it is your
own fat, there's no risk of allergic reactions as can occur with
other fillers. Unlike bovine collagen, the results may last for a
year or longer. Studies show that up to 80 percent of the injected fat may remain after one year, and that an average of
50 percent of the injection remains after two years.

One downside of autologous fat transfer is the extra step
of harvesting the fat from your body. If you're already undergoing a liposuction procedure, you can use some of the fat

from that process. However, in the majority of cases, people undergo a quick liposuction in the doctor's office of the area they've chosen for the harvest. This is an added cost to the procedure. Immediately after the fat is collected, it is processed and injected into the areas selected.

The average cost for an autologous fat transfer is $1,500 for harvest of the fat and one injection to the face and $150 to $450 per area for each additional touch-up treatment that uses fat harvested from the first procedure. Extra fat collected from your liposuction can be frozen and stored until you are ready to use it in later treatments. If, for some reason, sufficient fat is not saved from the first harvest, you will need to pay another liposuction fee before you have any additional injections.

Here's what you can expect if you choose to undergo autologous fat transfer:

- The doctor numbs the site you've chosen for the harvest, using a local anesthetic (diluted lidocaine). After the area is numb (this takes about 15 to 20 minutes), the fat is extracted through a pinhole using a hollow instrument called a cannula (like a skinny straw). The cannula is attached to a negative pressure syringe that gently removes from one-third of an ounce (10 cc) to a pint of fat, depending on the number and size of areas being treated.
- The harvested fat is centrifuged to remove the serum and oils, and the sample is washed and put into a syringe for the transplant.
- A topical anesthetic is applied over the wrinkles to be treated.

- The fat is slowly injected under the wrinkles to build up the area. The doctor must be careful not to inject too much fat, because the body will not be able to nourish the tissue, and the grafted fat may not "take."
- You will need to return for two more fat injections over the next six months. That's because fat does a funny thing: your body will absorb and dissipate more of the fat that is injected than it keeps at the injection site. In rare cases, the body absorbs the entire fat transfer. However, in most cases, about 70 percent of the first fat injection is absorbed. When you return for your next injections, a thin layer of fat will be added on top of the previous layer. Although you may be slightly swollen after each injection, the swelling usually disappears within 24 hours. The good news is that with enough fat removal, some of the fat harvested at the time of your first injection can be stored for your future injections.

AlloDerm

AlloDerm is the brand name of a soft, pliable implant that is made of human tissue (derived from tissue banks from human cadavers). It has an advantage over collagen and fat in that it can regenerate normal tissue in the implant area, which means it actually becomes a part of your body. This feature has a benefit, because the implant feels very natural (all wrinkle fillers look natural, but AlloDerm and fat *feel* natural), but it does not eliminate the need for another procedure sometime in the future. The implants are rarely permanent, and experts are not yet sure how long patients have to wait until they need another implant, because studies were not complete at the time of this writing.

In 1992, AlloDerm was developed to help burn victims and people who needed reconstructive surgery. Over the years, it has made its way into the cosmetic scene. It can be folded and manipulated to fill out wrinkles and other facial contours, and is especially helpful for laugh and marionette lines. It is not intended for fine lines.

Because it is an implant, the doctor will need to make a tiny incision, requiring only one or two sutures, to insert the material under the skin. The sutures can be removed in three to five days. There may be some bruising at the implant site, which you can cover with makeup. Swelling may last for a few days and can be relieved with an ice pack as needed. Some patients take an over-the-counter painkiller such as acctaminophcn or ibuprofcn to control any discomfort aftcr the procedure. The average cost for the entire procedure, per implant, is $2,000 to $3,000.

Cymetra

This injectable filler is made by the same company that makes AlloDerm, and similarly it consists of human tissue that has been donated to tissue banks in the United States. The tissue is treated and made into a dry powder (micronized) that is then mixed with solution and used as an injectable wrinkle filler (unlike AlloDerm, which is implanted). It is commonly used to reduce or eliminate marionette and laugh lines, and for lip augmentation.

One thing that separates this injectable from bovine collagen (besides the fact that it comes from your own species) is its ability to repopulate and restructure the skin once it has been injected. But as with collagen, you will need repeat injections to keep the look you want. That's because your body can absorb some of the injection over time. As with Allo-Derm, experts are not yet certain how long these injections last before you need another treatment. The average cost of each injection is $600 to $900.

Cymetra has several advantages. Because it actually becomes a part of your skin, it feels, looks, and ages like your own skin. And because it is not a foreign substance (even though it isn't your own tissue), there is very little risk that your body will reject it or that you will have an allergic reaction to it. That means you don't need to take an allergy test before getting the injection.

Doris was thrilled when her dermatologist told her about Cymetra. "I'd been wanting to do something about those terrible lines down the sides of my mouth," says the sixty-three-year-old retired teacher, "but I didn't want to get a face-lift. I was also not too enthused about collagen, so when I heard there was something made from human tissue, I thought I'd try it."

Doris went in for her injections at 9 in the morning and was out dancing that same evening. "There was a little bit of swelling, but I just put some ice on it, and it was barely noticeable by evening," she says. "It was gone by the next morning, and I've been happy ever since then. It's been eight months, and my face still looks great."

As with a Botox injection, you can choose to apply a topical anesthetic before the procedure, and your doctor can apply ice to the treatment site for a few minutes before the injection. Cymetra also contains a mild painkiller (lidocaine), which provides adequate pain relief for most people. Doris's experience with the procedure was typical, as most individuals return to their normal activities the same or the following day. Slight bruising or swelling may occur, but it usually disappears within six to twelve hours.

Expanded Polytetrafluoroethylene (ePTFE)

Expanded polytetrafluoroethylene (ePTFE) is a long name for what is commonly known as gortex, the same weather-resistant synthetic material found in some sportswear. For years, surgeons have used gortex as a suture material because it can be left permanently and safely inside the body. Several types of ePTFE implants are available, including Gore-Tex, SoftForm, and UltraSoft. These types of implants are similar, so we discuss them together. They are best as fillers for deep facial wrinkles, such as nasolabial creases and marionette lines. Their advantages are:

- An allergic reaction is extremely rare, because these inert fillers do not evoke an immune reaction within the body. This eliminates the need for an allergy test before the implant procedure, saving you both time and money.
- A local anesthetic is all you need when you have ePTFE implanted.
- They are permanent; they are not absorbed into the body.

Of course, there are disadvantages as well. These fillers are often implanted in the area of the mouth, so the real, albeit rare, potential for shifting and movement of the implant exists because of the great amount of activity associated with talking, chewing, and smiling. If an implant shifts, your doctor may need to remove and reposition it. Some other drawbacks include:

- There is a small risk (4 percent) of infection, so your doctor will likely put you on a short course of post-procedure antibiotics.
- Bruising and swelling tend to last a few days longer than you would experience with a collagen or fat injection.
- Placement of the implant requires a skilled doctor, because the material may be visible under the skin if not placed precisely. Make certain your doctor has experience in its use.

The average price for all of the ePTFE wrinkle fillers is $2,000 to $3,000 per implant.

CHEMICAL PEELS

How would you like to simply peel away lines and wrinkles like the outer skin of an onion and let a new, younger skin shine forth? That's the idea behind a chemical peel. The pH of the skin (a measurement of its acidity) is 5.5, which is slightly acidic. When you do a chemical peel, a chemical solution that has a different pH is applied to your skin, which causes irritation and a "burn." This burning process removes layers of skin, and as the skin heals, new, younger-looking skin, free of age spots, emerges.

"Chemical peels are one of the most flexible treatments to rejuvenate aging skin and erase the marks of sun damage and age," says Gary D. Monheit, MD, associate professor in the department of dermatology at the University of Alabama Medical Center in Birmingham. They are effective for fading or removing fine facial wrinkles. If the thought of putting chemicals on your face makes you hesitate, consider this: more than two million chemical peels are performed in the United States every year. And when they are done by a qualified professional, you can look forward to smoother skin with more even tone.

Various formulas can be used for chemical peels, but the potency and depth of the peel are more important than which chemicals are used, says Dr. Monheit. To determine which approach is best for you, your physician will evaluate your skin type, pigmentation, and the extent of sun damage, and talk to you about the areas of your skin where the chemical peels can help you. Only then can she or he choose the strength and depth of the chemical peel that's right for you.

Before You Peel

The best candidates for chemical peels are usually people who have fair skin. While a light peel is generally safe for all skin types, medium peels are usually not recommended for people who have highly pigmented skin, such as African-American, Latino, Asian, and Indian people, or for those who come from the Mediterranean region, because there is the possibility of hypopigmentation (lightening of the skin).

You are not a candidate for a chemical peel if you have preexisting dermatitis (any inflammatory skin condition, including inflamed acne) or any active infection of the face (e.g., herpes, candida) or a rash. Also, if you are ill (e.g., the flu, cold, bronchitis), you should wait until your illness has passed.

Because medium chemical peels penetrate below the top layer of skin and thus are more invasive than a light peel, there are some precautions that you will need to take to prevent complications. We discuss those precautions below, so you will be aware of them when you have your consultation with your doctor. (Deep chemical peels penetrate deeper into the skin than a medium peel, and thus can correct more severe lines and wrinkles. However, like laser resurfacing, deep peels involve one to two weeks of downtime, and for that reason, they are mentioned only briefly in this book.)

Pretreatment Guidelines for Medium Chemical Peels

Before you undergo a medium chemical peel, your doctor should discuss the following pretreatment guidelines with you.

- **Stop smoking.** You should stop smoking at least one week before and for several weeks after the procedure. Smoking robs the skin tissues of oxygen, which they need to heal. Stopping smoking is not critical for a light peel, but it is recommended.

- **Hold off on herbs.** At least one week before the procedure, you should stop taking any vitamin and herbal supplements, especially those that can thin the blood (e.g., St. John's wort, feverfew, ginkgo biloba, garlic). This precaution is recommended because very little is known about how herbs affect wound healing, says Dr. Sengelmann.

- **Pretreat your skin.** Many doctors ask their patients to pretreat their skin by using tretinoin (a vitamin A product such as Retin-A) or an alpha hydroxy acid cream (glycolic acid) for several weeks. This is a good practice, says Dr. Sengelmann. These products should be applied after the procedure as well, and pretreatment use gets patients into the habit of using them. However, she notes that there is no scientific basis for pretreating the skin with these products. Your doctor may also suggest you use a bleaching agent (hydroquinones), which can reduce the risk of discoloration. Once your skin heals from the procedure, your doctor will advise you to continue to use these products to help protect your skin and preserve the more youthful look you just paid for.

- Antiviral medication. You also will be asked to take a prescription antiviral medication, such as acyclovir or famciclovir (Zovirax). This is to help prevent an outbreak of herpes. "But I've never had herpes," you protest, "so why do I have to take an antiviral drug?" Chemical peels can activate a dormant herpes virus. Taking the drug is a precaution, but one you should comply with because if a herpes infection occurs after your treatment, you may get scarring. You will need to continue taking the antiviral medication for about ten days after your treatment as well.

Preparing for the Peel

The basic approach to each type of chemical peel is similar. If you are getting a light peel, an anesthetic isn't necessary. For a medium-depth peel, it may be helpful to use topical lidocaine or a lidocaine/prilocaine combination product. You can ask your doctor for a prescription or the name of over-the-counter brands. Another option is to take a relaxant or pain reliever before the peel (e.g., acetaminophen, ibuprofen). These are options you should discuss with your doctor.

The doctor will clean your face to remove dirt, soap, and oils. Then, using a swab applicator, the chemical will be applied to the selected areas of your face, or to your entire face if you've chosen a full-face peel. For medium peels, you may feel moderate burning and a tingling sensation for several minutes, followed by temporary throbbing that lasts about 5 to 10 minutes and is generally a 5 to 7 on a 10-point pain scale. Light peels may cause some slight tingling and burning.

Here are some things you should know about light and medium chemical peels. If you are thinking about getting a chemical peel, talk to your doctor about exactly how he or she does the procedure.

Light "Lunch-Time" Peel

The most popular and commonly performed chemical peel is the "lunch-time" peel, so named because it can be done in less than an hour, and you can return to work looking great. But quick and easy is a trade-off for what you get: a superficial peel that is a great way to fade freckles and give your face a glow, but is only minimally effective against fine lines and age spots. It also helps increase the production of collagen.

For a light peel, your doctor or cosmetologist will use either an alpha or beta hydroxy acid (naturally occurring compounds mostly derived from various types of fruits; see chapter 10), or an amino fruit acid peel, which consists of amino acids found in sugarcane. The most common acid used is glycolic acid, which is a type of alpha hydroxy acid. If you go to a spa or salon, the cosmetologist is allowed to use only a low concentration of glycolic acid (20 to 30 percent). Your doctor (or his or her nurse), however, can use a higher concentration (up to 70 percent).

For optimal results, sometimes up to six treatments are needed. At each treatment, the concentration of the peeling substance will be increased, and/or it will be left on your face longer. The treatments can be done once a week or at longer intervals. You should discuss the scheduling with your doctor. Some people, however, are completely satisfied with the results after only one or two treatments. Your level of satisfaction can depend on your skin type, the extent of your fine lines, and your expectations. Once the series is over, you may choose to return for repeat treatments months or years later, depending on how well you maintain your skin and how you feel about any age-related changes that are occurring on your face.

A possible negative side of a light peel is that some people experience skin irritation from alpha or beta hydroxy acids. If this happens to you, or you know you have sensitive skin, use an amino fruit acid peel instead. It is buffered by amino molecules, which makes it much less irritating, and it also enhances collagen production. The results are similar to those with a glycolic acid peel.

The average cost of a light chemical peel is $100 to $125 per treatment session.

Medium Peel

If you have fine lines and wrinkles and moderate sun damage, and you don't mind a little downtime, a medium-depth peel may be for you. Instead of the two to six treatments needed to achieve good results with a light chemical peel, you need to show up for only one in-office visit for a medium peel. This type of peel must be done by a doctor, who will use trichloracetic acid, or TCA, to selectively peel your skin to a certain level. New York dermatologist John F. Romano says he has women in their late sixties and seventies who really like the TCA peel. "It freshens up the face better than fruit peels or glycolic acid," he says. "If you have the time to hide away for a few days, it can really do a very nice job on light lines and wrinkles, removing sun damage, and brightening up the skin." After a downtime of five to seven days, the results can last for five years. You can expect to pay an average of $450 to $1,500 for a full-face peel.

When you leave your doctor's office after a medium peel, you won't need any bandages. You will, however, have a layer of petroleum jelly on the treated areas of your face, and you will need to reapply this often for a few days to protect your healing skin and to keep it moist. You will also continue to take any antiviral and antibiotic medication your doctor prescribed.

Side effects from a TCA peel, which can include prolonged redness, hyperpigmentation (darkening of the skin), hypopigmentation (lightening of the skin), or scarring, are rare. You can best avoid these problems by going to a qualified physician for your TCA treatment.

Regardless of the type of chemical peel you get, an essential part of the treatment program is ongoing use of sunscreen and daily skin care, including the use of topical alpha hydroxy, vitamin A derivatives, and bleaching creams (see chapter 10). Your doctor will discuss the specific ingredients and products that are most beneficial for you.

MICRODERMABRASION

The term "microdermabrasion" refers to a procedure in which super-fine aluminum oxide crystals are sprayed onto the skin and then removed with a vacuum-like device. As the crystals are vacuumed up, they whirl around on the top layer of skin and perform a very fine sanding effect, which removes fine lines and wrinkles, reduces brown spots, stimulates collagen production, and leaves behind softer, younger-looking skin. Microdermabrasion is a variation on dermabrasion, a more invasive procedure that uses a sanding device to penetrate into the second layer of skin, or dermis.

"It's like getting your face polished," says Toni, a forty-nine-year-old grandmother who underwent microdermabrasion. "When my grandchild asked why my face was cracked and crinkled, I laughed, but I wasn't amused. The very next day I made an appointment with my doctor and told him to sand away the fine wrinkles on my checks, the crow's-feet near my eyes, and the lines above my lips."

Like light chemical peels, microdermabrasion requires a series of treatments, usually two to six, to get optimal results. Treatments are only mildly uncomfortable—some people describe feeling a slight stinging sensation. The treatments can be done as often as once a week, but three- or four-week intervals are common. Each treatment takes about 20 to 45 minutes, depending on the number of areas treated. Treatments are generally done by a qualified nurse or medical assistant.

You can return to work or other activities immediately after each treatment, with a fresh pink glow to your face. Your doctor will likely advise you to use topical vitamin A or alpha hydroxy products daily to help maintain your results, as well as sunscreen. The average cost per microdermabrasion treatment is $75 to $300, depending on the amount of area treated.

NON-ABLATIVE LASER

Jessica, a forty-five-year-old sales manager, flipped open her hand-held computer and checked off the rest of her tasks and appointments for the day: "Sales meeting at 2 o'clock, pick up dry cleaning after meeting, laser treatment of face at 5:30, meet Steve for dinner at 7 o'clock."

Was Jessica going to dinner with a bag over her head? How could she have a laser treatment at 5:30 and be presentable for dinner just over an hour later? Because Jessica was having a non-ablative laser treatment, the "lunch-time laser" that is quickly growing in popularity.

"Non-ablative lasers are very popular because people don't want downtime," says Dr. Jaliman. Unlike traditional lasers, which use heat to remove the top skin tissue, non-ablative laser treatments penetrate the top layer of skin, or epidermis, without leaving any telltale signs of redness or irritation to the skin's outer layer. Instead, the laser beams enter the dermis, where blood vessels and collagen reside, to do their work. Non-ablative laser treatments are good for removing fine lines, but not deep lines or wrinkles. Best results are seen with crow's-feet and wrinkles between the eyebrows (frown lines).

Several non-ablative lasers are currently on the market, including NLite, Cool Touch, Smooth Beam, and V Beam, among others. All work similarly: all cool the epidermis to provide comfort and protection to the skin while the lasers penetrate into the dermis to cause collagen remodeling.

The Procedure
Each non-ablative laser treatment takes about 15 to 20 minutes, is done in your doctor's office, and is painless, so

no anesthesia is needed. Your eyes will be covered with goggles to protect them during the treatment. Your doctor will direct the laser and deliver a series of yellow, red, or infrared beams that pass into the dermis and reach the red blood cells and pigment cells. These cells absorb the yellow and red light, break apart, and are absorbed by the body's healing process. The infrared beam stimulates the production of new collagen beneath the wrinkles and thus plumps out the skin.

After a series of up to six treatments about one month apart, says Dr. Jaliman, you have new collagen and smoother, younger-looking skin, all without any visible injury to the skin. Another advantage of this laser approach is that the doctor can fine-tune the rays to meet your specific skin condition and type. You must practice a little patience with this technique, however. Don't expect to see a lot of improvement in your skin until about the third treatment, which is when collagen production peaks. Even before then, however, you should see some improvement.

Once you get the look you want, you may need further treatments every three to six months to maintain that look. Generally, the older you are, the less responsive your skin will be to the laser, and the more often you may need treatments. But if you're careful about protecting yourself against the sun's rays, your results will last longer.

After each treatment, you must protect your skin from the sun by applying sunscreen of at least 15 SPF. Some people report some minor redness and swelling for a few hours or pinpoint bruising that can last up to a week. This can easily be covered with makeup.

Combining Non-Ablative with Other Procedures

Some doctors are using Botox injections along with non-ablative laser treatments to treat fine lines around the eyes and mouth. When low doses of Botox are carefully injected around the mouth and eyes, they can enhance the results of the laser treatment. Others are combining the laser treatment with collagen injections to eliminate wrinkles in the forehead and around the mouth and nose.

"Some doctors are combining non-ablative laser with erbium laser (an invasive laser procedure that involves a week of downtime) and those results seem better," says New York dermatologist John F. Romano, who believes the results with non-ablative laser are subtle at best when used alone. "Non-ablative laser treatments are expensive," he says, "about $500 per treatment area, but they're popular because there's no downtime." Non-ablative laser can also be used following chemical peels, microdermabrasion, or face-lifts to enhance the results.

MORE INVASIVE COSMETIC PROCEDURES

This chapter has focused on cosmetic procedures that are associated with no or minimal downtime, which are the types of skin enhancement that appeal to the majority of women. However, we wanted to mention a few other procedures that are sometimes used along with Botox injections but that involve days or weeks of healing. The explanations for these approaches are intentionally brief; therefore, if you are interested in any of them, you will want to discuss them in more detail with your physician.

Laser Resurfacing

Laser resurfacing has been described as a very precisely controlled injury to the skin that can remove 50 to 70 percent of wrinkles. The laser removes the top layer of skin and penetrates into the dermis to heat up and intentionally damage the collagen. The damage is beneficial, because the healing process results in the formation of new collagen, which, over the next few months, results in tighter, smoother skin. During the first 7 to 10 days after treatment, however, your skin will be very tender, red, and oozing.

Because laser resurfacing is an invasive procedure, you will need to take antiviral medication before and after the procedure (see "Chemical Peels"). Your doctor will likely prescribe an antibiotic as well, as there is a risk of wound infection. For the laser treatment itself, you will need an injectable anesthetic (such as lidocaine) and an oral relaxant, or possibly an intravenous sedative or general anesthesia. After the treatment, you may need painkillers for the discomfort and ice packs to relieve the swelling. The doctor will apply ointments or dressing to help keep your skin moist and protected, and you must reapply these for up to ten days until your new epidermis forms.

Risks of laser resurfacing include scarring, temporary darkening of the skin, or permanent lightening of the skin. Dry, tight skin is a side effect of this procedure. The average cost of laser resurfacing is $1,500 to $7,000, depending on how much of the face is treated.

Radio Frequency Ablation

Radio frequency is a type of non-ablative laser procedure that involves minimal downtime. Also known as cold ablation, this approach delivers energy to the dermis without affecting the epidermis. The best candidates are people who have severe photo damage and deep wrinkles.

A topical anesthetic cream is applied before treatment begins. Radio frequency energy is absorbed by the collagen, stimulating new production. Treatment takes about 15 to 30 minutes and costs an average of $3,000. After the treatment, your doctor will prescribe an ointment to keep your skin moist, and you may need to wear bandages for a day or two. The treated skin may be swollen for up to three to four days, sometimes longer if you were treated around the eyes. New skin will grow back in about one week, and the initial redness from the treatment will gradually fade to pink, which may remain for several weeks or months.

Dermabrasion

The term "dermabrasion" refers to a procedure in which a very high-speed rotating sanding brush or wheel is used to remove layers of skin, and with it, wrinkles, acne scars, and other skin imperfections. Because dermabrasion removes the epidermis and reaches the lower layer of skin, it allows new skin cells to move up quickly to the top layer during healing, resulting in smoother, younger-looking skin. Pre- and post-treatment precautions are needed, including the use of antiviral and antibiotic medications (see "Chemical Peels," page 142). For the procedure itself, you will receive a local anesthetic. After the procedure, your doctor will apply bandages, which you can remove in a day or two. Your skin will slowly heal over the next five to eight days. Risks include temporary darkening of the skin, permanent lightening of the skin, or scarring. The average cost is $1,500 to $3, 500, depending on the area(s) treated.

Deep Chemical Peel (Phenol)

The procedure for a deep chemical peel is similar to that for a medium peel (see "Chemical Peels"), except the chemical used, typically phenol, is more powerful. For this reason, it is important to be treated by a physician with experience and in a controlled environment (in which there is heart monitoring and resuscitation equipment, as there is a risk of arrhythmia—irregular rhythm of the heart).

The advantages of a phenol peel are that the entire process is done in one visit, the effects are usually dramatic and very satisfying (especially if you have deep wrinkles), and they are essentially permanent. The cost for these advantages is an average of $3,000 to $5,000. The downtime, however, is significant: at least two weeks to heal to a point where you will feel comfortable appearing in public. You will need to wear bandages for at least several days following treatment. After about seven days, new skin will form, but it will remain red and peeling for a month or more.

Phenol is very toxic to the cells responsible for your skin's pigmentation, and many patients experience a permanent lightening of the skin from a phenol peel. That's why the ideal candidate for a phenol peel is someone who already has very light skin.

QUESTIONS AND ANSWERS

One of the salons in my area advertises chemical peels. Is it safe to get it at a salon or spa?

There's nothing wrong with getting a "lunch-time" or light chemical peel or a fruit peel at a spa or salon if it is done by a licensed cosmetologist or aesthetician and you know the facility is equipped to handle any complications that may arise (e.g., there should be a dermatologist on call). A light chemical peel at a spa or salon is usually less expensive than one done by a physician, and you may get some pampering along with the peel. However, you should also explore the possibility of having your light peel done by a physician and compare the costs, convenience, and safety factors before making a decision.

Remember that doctor-supervised peels are allowed to reach much higher concentrations of acid (up to 70 percent versus up to only 30 percent in a spa or salon). Therefore, a light chemical peel done by a doctor can produce better results. Even when higher concentrations of acid are used, however, the results will not be like those achieved with a medium chemical peel.

You should also know that in some states, having a medical degree is not required to do a chemical peel, including medium and deep peels. You can check with your state's health department for the requirements in your area. For your own safety, however, you should have a medium or deep peel performed by a qualified doctor only.

I'm concerned about using any injection or implant that comes from human tissue. How do I know I won't get a transmittable disease from the procedure?

The United States Tissue Bank has a very comprehensive process that it uses to screen all donated tissue. All samples are carefully tested and certified according to criteria established by the Food and Drug Administration. The freeze-drying process that is used removes all the cells from the tissue samples and leaves only the structural components, including collagen and elastin. All samples must be free of hepatitis B and C, human immunodeficiency virus (HIV), and syphilis, and all samples are examined after processing to make sure they have not been contaminated anywhere along the way. There has never been a reported case of infection from hepatitis, HIV, or syphilis from injection or implantation of products made from these tissues.

I heard about a new wrinkle filler called Artecol. Is it effective, and where can I get it?

Artecol consists of a mixture of bovine collagen and micronized plastic beads, and it is being used in Europe. After Artecol is injected, the bovine collagen is slowly absorbed over time. This leaves the plastic beads behind, which help keep the wrinkles from returning. Reports from Europe claim that the beads remain in the area permanently. This form of wrinkle filler has not been approved in the United States by the Food and Drug Administration (FDA).

What is hyaluronic acid? I heard it can be used to fill out wrinkles.

Hyaluronic acid is a natural substance found in human skin. That's one feature that makes it a logical choice for injection into the skin to eliminate wrinkles. For now, it is being used in Europe and Canada and has not been approved for use in the United States. If you've seen or heard the names Perlane, Restylane, or Hylaform, those are brands of hyaluronic acid. There are attempts being made to have hyaluronic acid approved for use in the United States.

Like collagen, hyaluronic acid injections must be repeated every four to six months to keep the wrinkles away. Different formulations work well for fine versus deep wrinkles, as is the case with bovine collagen. The side effects are similar to those seen with bovine collagen, with a significantly lower incidence of allergy expected.

I'd like to get rid of my laugh lines, because they look awful. What's the best way to eliminate these creases?

Laugh lines are often best eliminated using one of several different types of wrinkle fillers, such as bovine collagen, fat, a human tissue product, or a permanent implant. Some people find that microdermabrasion or non-ablative laser treatment along with the wrinkle fillers provides a more pleasing result. Talk to your doctor about your options.

My crow's-feet are so bad I usually wear sunglasses to hide them. What's the best way to get rid of these wrinkles?

You will need to discuss your options with your doctor. However, popular options include Botox injections alone, laser resurfacing alone, or Botox combined with laser resurfacing, chemical peels, or a filler such as bovine collagen. If your crow's-feet are pronounced, your doctor may recommend a combination approach. That's because while laser resurfacing can eliminate much of the wrinkling, you will likely still continue to smile and crinkle the skin around your eyes. Botox injections can relax the muscles responsible for creating those lines and greatly enhance your laser treatment.

What kind of precautions do I need to take after getting a bovine collagen injection?

Virtually none. There's no downtime associated with bovine collagen injections. You're free to wear makeup, eat, and drink after treatment. Some people experience some mild swelling and redness, which typically disappears in several hours to a day. If these symptoms persist, contact your doctor.

I'm thinking about getting a full-face laser resurfacing treatment for my lines and wrinkles and some brown spots. Will I need to go into the hospital for this? Isn't there some risk involved with this procedure?

Most doctors perform these procedures in their office; however, some use hospital outpatient facilities. Talk to your doctor about where he does his treatments.

People who undergo a full-face laser treatment often get intravenous sedation (sometimes called twilight sleep or conscious sedation) or, in some cases, general anesthesia. These levels of sedation must be monitored by a certified registered nurse or a physician anesthesiologist. Because there are added risks associated with conscious sedation and general anesthesia, your doctor must have emergency equipment and trained staff available in the rare case you would require cardiopulmonary resuscitation.

These cautions are mentioned not to scare you but to alert you to the possible risks. However, some dermatologic surgeons do the entire procedure with the patient fully awake and comfortable using local anesthesia and nerve blocks (e.g., lidocaine), in addition to relaxants taken orally. If you choose to have general anesthesia for your procedure, you will be required to undergo preoperative testing (including blood tests and usually a chest x-ray and an electrocardiogram [EKG]) before your laser procedure and have preoperative clearance from your primary doctor to ensure you are in good health.

Is there a relationship between getting collagen injections and connective tissue disease or autoimmune disease?

There have been reports of cases of connective tissue disease (e.g., rheumatoid arthritis, dermatomyositis, systemic lupus erythematosus, and polymyositis, which are all autoimmune diseases) developing in people after they received bovine collagen injections. The cases appeared in individuals who had no previous history of these medical conditions. Experts have not established that the injections were the cause of these diseases, and there is no reason to suspect this was more than coincidental development of disease. However, if you already have a connective tissue disease, you should talk to your doctor before getting bovine collagen injections. Your doctor will likely advise you to choose another wrinkle filler.

10

CARING FOR YOUR SKIN,
FROM THE INSIDE OUT
AND THE OUTSIDE IN

IF YOU WANT to keep your skin looking its best, which includes eliminating or reducing wrinkles and sun damage, you need to nurture it from the inside as well as the outside. Earlier in this book we talked about the major impact sun exposure has on your skin and ways you can minimize the damage—the fine lines, wrinkles, brown spots, changes in pigmentation, and the broken blood vessels—it can cause. We told you not to smoke, to get enough sleep, to avoid environmental pollutants, and to minimize stress.

But we haven't said much about how you can nourish and pamper your skin. Your skin is a vital, living organ—the largest organ of the human body—and it needs to be fed and cared for every day. The skin that people usually see first is your face, and so you want it to look its very best at all times.

Skin care and wrinkle prevention require more than just hiding from the sun; they include attention to the food you eat, the supplements you take, and the products you put on your skin—"cosmeceuticals," a term used to describe topical cosmetic products that reportedly have medicinal properties that enhance the beauty and health of the skin. Therefore, in this chapter we explore each of these areas and explain what works and does not work when it comes to keeping your skin as fresh, young, and wrinkle-free and skin-cancer–free as possible.

DOES WHAT YOU EAT MATTER?

Because food and eating are a big part of our lives, the eternal question "How much does what we eat matter to our health?" is one that scientists as well as the general public ask frequently. The connection between diet and wrinkles has been specifically examined.

The *Journal of the American College of Nutrition* (2001) contained one such connection recorded by a group of researchers. They noticed that when they looked collectively at the elderly people in various countries, regardless of whether the people had light or dark skin, some were less likely than others to get wrinkles. The scientists were curious about this, so they decided to look at what the people were eating to see if they could find a relationship between diet and the development and presence of wrinkles.

The researchers measured the wrinkles and examined the eating habits of more than 450 men and women aged 70 and older who were living in Australia, Greece, and Sweden. After they analyzed the foods consumed by the participants in each country, they noted the following:

- Greeks who ate large amounts of beans and green leafy vegetables had fewer wrinkles than Greeks who ate high-fat foods, such as pudding, butter, and processed meats.

- Australians who ate asparagus, melons, multigrain breads, tea, grapes, and sardines had fewer wrinkles than those who ate sugary foods (desserts), meats, and dairy foods.

- Swedes who focused on low-fat dairy foods, lima beans, and spinach pie fared better when it came to wrinkles than their countrymen who ate ice cream, red meat, fried potatoes, and soft drinks.

Overall, the researchers found that people who ate more vegetables, fish, beans, peas, and low-fat dairy products had much less skin damage and wrinkling than people who consumed fatty dairy foods, red meats, and foods that contain a lot of sugar. They also noted that foods rich in vitamin C, calcium, magnesium, phosphorus, iron, and zinc seemed to protect the skin from wrinkles.

Do these findings sound vaguely familiar? We're often told that eating fruits and vegetables (at least five servings daily, preferably more), choosing low-fat dairy products rather than full-fat varieties, avoiding red meat when possible, eating more fish, selecting whole grains and cereals, including beans and some soy in our diets, avoiding sugary foods, and drinking six to eight glasses of pure water a day are all tips that can help us prevent a host of diseases and maintain good health.

This is also sound nutritional advice if you want healthy skin and you want to slow down the aging process. Experts have broken down this advice for us and identified which specific components in these foods are most helpful when it comes to maintaining youthful, healthy skin. Let's look at some of those components here.

EATING FOR HEALTHY SKIN

Every time you have a meal or a snack, you could be contributing to your skin's health and reducing the advancement of wrinkles. The trouble is, you must first know which foods contain the nutrients that are most beneficial for your skin. Key nutrients for skin health include antioxidants, B vitamins, and protein, as well as fiber, water, and fats. We've brought those foods and nutrients together for you here.

Antioxidants

Antioxidants are a group of special vitamins, minerals, and other nutrients that help fight free radicals and the damage they can cause to your skin cells. Free radicals are renegade molecules that are set into action in many ways, and one of those ways is exposure to the sun. When the sun's ultraviolet rays penetrate your dermis, they stimulate free-radical production and activity. The more sun exposure you have, the more free-radical activity there is. As more and more free radicals are created, they damage your healthy skin cells, collagen, and elastin, which accelerates the aging process and causes wrinkles to form.

Getting enough antioxidants in your diet can be easy if you eat at least five servings of fruits and vegetables daily (while deep-fried onion rings and French fries are vegetables, they are not a good choice because they are fried). Other good sources of antioxidants are legumes (e.g., beans, lentils, peas) and whole grains and cereals; eat six to eleven servings of these foods daily.

The antioxidants most commonly associated with skin health are vitamins A (usually consumed in the form of beta-carotene), C, and E, the minerals selenium, zinc, and copper, and the nutrient coenzyme Q10. Here's why these antioxidants are so helpful to the skin, and which foods to include in your diet in order to enjoy their benefits.

Vitamin A (beta-carotene). We often hear about the benefits of vitamin A when it's applied topically to the skin (more on that below), but getting it in your diet also helps your skin. Vitamin A is helpful with wound healing, which is especially important if you are recovering from dermabrasion, a chemical peel, or laser resurfacing.

Because vitamin A is a fat-soluble vitamin, appropriate dosing is important. An overabundance of ingested vitamin A can accumulate in the body and become toxic, causing symptoms like headache, scaly skin, nausea, and diarrhea. That's why it's better to take its precursor, beta-carotene, which converts to vitamin A once it's in the body. Because beta-carotene is water-soluble, it does not get stored in the body and therefore it is not toxic.

Rich sources of beta-carotene are typically orange and green fruits and vegetables, including apricots, broccoli, cantaloupe, carrots, kale, pumpkin, spinach, squash, and sweet potatoes.

Vitamin C. This vitamin, also known as ascorbic acid, is critical for skin health not only because it fights free radicals, but because it helps to produce collagen. It also plays a role in wound healing and strengthening the walls of your blood vessels.

This water-soluble vitamin needs to be replenished every day. You can keep your body well supplied with vitamin C by making these foods a part of your daily diet: berries, broccoli, Brussels sprouts, cabbage, cauliflower, grapefruit, guava, kale, lemons, oranges, pepper, spinach, strawberries, and tomatoes.

Vitamin E. It's been shown that low levels of vitamin E in the body are associated with acne, which indicates that it has benefits for the skin. This fat-soluble vitamin helps protect your body's cells from free-radical damage and also stabilizes vitamin A and C. You'll get vitamin E when you eat almonds, filberts, walnuts, wheat germ, whole-grain flours, and oils (corn, olive, peanut, safflower, sunflower, wheat germ).

Selenium. This mineral works with vitamin E to help prevent free-radical damage to tissues, and thus it can help slow the aging process. It also appears to play a role in repairing damaged cells. You can enjoy selenium in the following foods: barley, broccoli, cabbage, celery, cucumbers, garlic, mushrooms, onions, wheat germ, and whole-grain flours.

Zinc and Copper. We talk about these two minerals together because they work hand-in-hand to neutralize free radicals and protect your body's cell membranes against free-radical damage. Zinc is also critical for keeping your immune system operating at its best. Both zinc and copper are instrumental in wound healing, which makes them especially important if you undergo a cosmetic procedure such as a medium chemical peel.

Good sources of zinc include garlic, whole grains, soybeans, sunflower seeds, blackstrap molasses, wheat germ, mushrooms, and eggs. You'll find copper in barley, lentils, blackstrap molasses, mushrooms, oatmeal, nuts, and wheat germ.

Coenzyme Q10. This vitamin-like substance is also known as ubiquinone, a term from the word "ubiquitous," which reveals that it is found in nearly all the cells in the body. Coenzyme Q10 is a potent antioxidant, which makes it helpful in maintaining skin health, and a main player in transforming food into a form that the body can use for energy.

Coenzyme Q10 is not found in many foods; thus, supplements are sometimes recommended (see below). Mackerel, peanuts, salmon, sardines, and spinach contain a good amount of this substance.

B Vitamins

The B vitamins work together in many different chemical reactions that protect the skin. For example, vitamin B_1 works with vitamin B_6 and vitamin E to neutralize free radicals. All of the B vitamins play a role in keeping the immune system healthy, and a healthy immune system is essential for healthy skin. Keeping your immune system in optimal shape can help promote healing of the skin, especially after procedures such as chemical peels and laser resurfacing, which have an associated risk of wound infection.

To help you eat your Bs, here are some excellent food sources:

- B_1 (thiamin): brown rice, chickpeas, navy beans, soybeans, wheat germ, whole-grain flours
- B_2 (riboflavin): almonds, black-eyed peas, wheat germ
- B_3 (niacin): beets, peanuts, sunflower seeds, brewer's yeast
- B_5 (pantothenic acid): corn, lentils, peanuts, peas, soybeans, sunflower seeds, whole-grain flours

- B_6 (pyridoxine): avocados, bananas, brown rice, carrots, lentils, soybeans, sunflower seeds, wheat germ, whole-grain flours
- B_{12} (cobalamin): liver, B_{12}-enriched cereals, dairy products
- Folic acid: barley, beans, brown rice, most fruits, green leafy vegetables, lentils, peas, soybeans, sprouts

Protein

Protein is a mixture of amino acids and is a critical part of the diet. Because protein is needed to help build and repair cells and tissues, including the skin, a low-protein diet can hinder this process. Although many people eat more than enough protein, individuals who are on diets often do not. "Enough" protein can be determined this way: 0.38 grams of protein per pound of body weight. Therefore, if you weigh 125 pounds, your daily intake of protein should be 47.5 grams. If you are very active, your need will be slightly higher. If you include a few ounces of protein at each meal (e.g., low-fat tofu, fish, skinless chicken, legumes) you should meet your goal. For her patients, Dr. Baumann recommends soy protein (tofu, soy milk, tempeh, soybeans) whenever possible.

Other Dietary Tips

Here are some other guidelines to consider when eating for healthier skin:

- Fiber: fiber helps keep your body and thus your skin hydrated, which keeps it looking its best. If you're eating lots of fruits, vegetables, and grains, you're probably getting a good supply of fiber. The recommended amount of daily fiber intake is 25 to 30 grams. Look for the words "100 percent whole wheat" on breads, rolls, and pasta.

- Water: six to eight 8-ounce glasses of pure water per day helps keep your skin hydrated. Keep a water bottle with you during the day and keep refilling it to remind yourself to drink.

- Fats: healthy fats, which include monounsaturated and some polyunsaturated fats, are important for healthy skin. Of course, use them in moderation. Experts generally recommend that 20 percent of your daily caloric intake be fat calories. Examples of healthy fats: monounsaturated fats include olives, olive oil, peanuts, avocado, and peanut oil; polyunsaturated fats include salmon, soybean oil, safflower oil, and walnuts. Examples of fats to avoid include margarine (and products containing hydrogenated or partially hydrogenated oils), butter, corn oil, coconut oils (in processed foods), whole milk and whole milk products, and animal fat in meats.

SUPPLEMENTATION

Although the optimal way for everyone to get their vitamins, minerals, and antioxidants is through their food, the reality is that most people don't always eat a nutritious diet. They have coffee and a doughnut for breakfast, skip lunch, work late and then stop at a fast-food restaurant on the way home, or pop a fat-laden frozen dinner into the microwave because they're too tired to cook. They're getting calories, but are they getting nutrition?

Why You Need Supplementation

Even if you have good intentions, the food you eat may not always be fresh, or it may be prepared in ways that rob it of its nutritional value. Lightly steaming, microwaving, or quickly stir-frying vegetables, for example, are good ways to retain their nutrients; overcooking them or deep-frying them are not. The addition of preservatives, artificial flavorings and colorings, and other additives to foods during processing can damage nutrients. Also try to avoid using pre-cut fruits and vegetables: they may be convenient, but because they have been cut and packaged, they lose a lot of their nutritional value. With all these strikes working against you, it helps to take high-potency nutritional supplements to keep you on track with your overall nutrition.

When shopping for a good vitamin or mineral supplement, you need to have an idea of how much of each nutrient you should be taking. One yardstick has been the Recommended Dietary Allowance (RDA), which was established to provide guidelines for the minimum nutritional needs for healthy individuals. (Note: In 1997, the Food and Nutrition Board of the National Research Council created the term *dietary reference intakes*, or DRIs, to replace the RDAs. This new term encompasses all the nutrients assigned an RDA value, plus some additional ones.)

Most experts agree that the majority of the DRI dosages fall far short of the amounts needed for people to maintain good health. The DRI for vitamin C, for example, is only

60 mg (200 mg for smokers), yet doctors routinely recommend dosages that are ten times that amount or higher.

How much of each nutrient does your body need? Not all doctors agree on the optimal dosages of nutrients to supplement your diet, but there are some general ranges that are recommended. As a guide, we offer the following list of suggested optimal dosages of supplements. You will need to take more than one supplement to meet these amounts—for example, a high-potency vitamin-mineral supplement, a balanced B-complex supplement, and a calcium supplement. (A supplement that contained all these amounts would be too big to swallow.) As always, you should check with a health-care provider who is knowledgeable about nutrition before starting a supplement program. Remember: more is not always better, especially when it comes to the fat-soluble vitamins, such as vitamins A, D, E, and K. Follow your doctor's advice on dosages.

- Beta-carotene: 25,000 IU
- Vitamin C: 100–1,000 mg
- Vitamin D: 100–400 IU
- Vitamin E: 400–800 IU
- Vitamin K: 60–300 mcg
- Vitamin B_1: 10–100 mg
- Vitamin B_2: 10–50 mg
- Vitamin B_3: 10–30 mg as niacinamide, to avoid the facial and body flush that accompanies niacin
- Vitamin B_5: 25–100 mg
- Vitamin B_6: 25–100 mg
- Folic acid: 400–800 mcg
- Vitamin B_{12}: 200–400 mcg
- Calcium: 800–1,200 mg

- Copper: 1–2 mg
- Zinc: 15–45 mg
- Magnesium: 250–500 mg
- Manganese: 10–15 mg
- Selenium: 100–200 mcg
- Potassium: 200–500 mg
- Coenzyme Q10: 30–100 mg

TREATING YOUR SKIN FROM
THE OUTSIDE IN

Just because a certain nutrient is beneficial for the skin when you take it orally, it doesn't necessarily follow that applying that same nutrient topically to the skin will produce the same results, or even any significant benefits at all. In this section, we help you choose the items that most benefit your skin from the outside in and tell you why they do work, may work, or don't work at all.

"I think it's very confusing for the general public to figure out what is good and what is not good for their skin, to separate what's hype from what's science," says Dr. Sengelmann. "When people read something in a beauty magazine, they take it for the truth. It can be hard to separate the marketing gimmicks from the facts." We hope what follows helps you find some of that truth for yourself.

Cosmeceuticals

Cosmeceuticals—skin-care products that manufacturers claim have therapeutic properties to improve the skin's beauty and health—are a mainstay of the beauty industry. They are sold everywhere: department stores, doctors' offices, drugstores, over the Internet, in catalogs, and at parties. Many claims have been made about how different topical products, including vitamin A (tretinoin, which is the topical form of the vitamin), vitamin C, vitamin E, alpha lipoic acid, copper peptides, coenzyme Q10, as well as other substances, such as alpha and beta hydroxy acids, collagen, elastin, and placenta, can help you look younger, eliminate wrinkles, and fight the effects of aging. You've probably seen dozens of skin-care products that advertise having one or more of these ingredients.

Which of these substances really help the skin when they are applied topically? What are their side effects? Are you just wasting your money if you buy products that contain these ingredients? When a product does contain an effective ingredient, does it contain enough to *be* effective? Should you just use soap on your face instead?

Here are some of the most common ingredients found in skin-care products and what the research says about them. First we talk about the most researched and arguably the most effective ingredients—alpha hydroxy and beta hydroxy acids, and tretinoin (vitamin A). We then turn to other ingredients you will often see in cosmetic products that may or may not be helpful. These are listed alphabetically and therefore their order in no way suggests that one is better or worse than another.

Investigations into the effectiveness of most of these ingredients are ongoing. New findings are being reported all the time, so you must weigh the results of these studies as they are published and decide whether a particular ingredient is right for you. Seek advice from a trusted dermatologist or other physician who is knowledgeable about skin care to help you make your selections.

After you learn about individual ingredients, we turn to a discussion of the three basic products you need for routine skin care: cleanser, moisturizer, and sunscreen. (We don't cover sunscreen in detail because it was discussed in chapter 3, but we mention it again to remind you how important it is for healthy, younger-looking skin.)

Alpha Hydroxy Acids

Alpha hydroxy acids (AHAs) are the largest category of cosmeceuticals on the market. Among the various AHAs that are available, glycolic acid, which is derived from sugarcane, is most commonly used because it has small molecules that can penetrate the skin, and is well adapted for cosmetic use. It is also one of the acids commonly used for light chemical peels (see chapter 9), although the concentration used in peels is greater than that used in skin-care products. Other AHAs include citric (from citrus fruits), lactic (sour milk), malic (apples), and tartaric (fruit and grape wine). Lactic acid is also used in many skin-care products.

Products containing alpha hydroxy acids, such as cleansers and lotions, are available over the counter and have proven to be helpful in enhancing the skin, depending on the strength of the product. They can remove layers of dead skin, help keep the skin hydrated, and increase the number of elastin fibers, which helps prevent wrinkling. The more concentrated products need to be purchased through your physician.

The products you'll find over the counter will contain less than a 10 percent concentration of alpha hydroxy acid and have a pH of 3.0 to 5.0. These values have been deemed safe and somewhat effective for daily use. Products used in salons and spas can contain a concentration of up to 30 percent. At this concentration, the products are only for brief, discontinuous use and can be applied only by professionals. Personnel under a physician's supervision are allowed to use AHAs with up to a 70 percent concentration, which will bring about the most dramatic results.

Although topical AHAs with a pH at the lower end of the range (and thus more acidic) are more effective, they also are more likely to irritate the skin. A product with a higher pH (more alkaline) will be milder, but somewhat less effective. Slight tingling and minor irritation can occur during the first two weeks of use. If it continues, or if you experience severe redness or irritation, stop using the product and consult your dermatologist.

Beta Hydroxy Acids

Beta hydroxy acids are similar to glycolic acid (one of the alpha hydroxy acids) because they enhance the skin's appearance by helping remove the dead skin layer from the epidermis. The most common beta hydroxy acid is salicylic acid, which is derived from the bark of willow trees, wintergreen leaves, and sweet birch bark. (If you recognize the name "salicylic," that's because it's an ingredient in aspirin, an anti-inflammatory drug.) Salicylic acid has been used for thousands of years to treat various skin conditions. The advantage of the beta hydroxy acids is that they are less irritating than the alpha hydroxy acids, and so are preferred by people who have sensitive skin.

Vitamin A

The advantages of vitamin A and its derivatives in improving the appearance of your skin have been well docu-

mented. Both the natural and the synthetic derivatives of vitamin A, which include tretinoin (retinoic acid), tazarotene,
retinol, and retinyl palmitrate, are known collectively as
retinoids. One of the better-recognized vitamin A–based
products is Retin-A, a prescription product that contains the
active ingredient tretinoin and has been used to treat acne
and wrinkles for more than fifteen years.

Prescription Vitamin A Products. Studies have proven
that tretinoin can reduce wrinkles and improve skin texture
and pigmentation. These benefits result from tretinoin's ability
to increase collagen in the dermis, reduce the amount of damaged elastin, and decrease the pigment melanin. The downsides: tretinoin is available only by prescription (Retin-A,
Retin-A Micro, Renova, Avita), and it can be very irritating to
the skin, causing redness and flaking as well as increased sun
sensitivity. Some vitamin A products contain moisturizers that
reduce these side effects.

Tazarotene is the latest addition to the retinoid group and
is available by prescription only. In a study conducted at the
University of Michigan Medical Center in Ann Arbor, researchers tested tazarotene cream against tretinoin cream in
349 patients. They found that tazarotene cream 0.1 percent
and tretinoin cream 0.05 percent were nearly equally effective at reducing fine wrinkles after 12 weeks of use. Overall,
however, participants who used tazarotene had more significant improvement in skin appearance after 8 weeks than people who were using tretinoin. Tazarotene has similar side
effects (sun sensitivity, flaking, irritation) as tretinoin.

Over-the-Counter Vitamin A Products. If you want the
benefits of vitamin A in over-the-counter (OTC) products,
look for those that contain retinol, as opposed to retinyl

palmitate, which does not appear to be active when applied on the skin. Retinol is converted to retinoic acid by the skin, and while it is less effective than tretinoin, it is also less irritating. Retinol is found in many moisturizers.

In order to remain effective, retinol must be combined with an antioxidant or another substance that resists breakdown when exposed to light, because retinol becomes unstable in light. In a study published in 2002, researchers found that a combination of retinol and salicylic acid (as discussed above, a beta hydroxy acid, and a relative of aspirin, it fights inflammation) reduced signs of photo aging after only three weeks of use. The participants reported an improvement in fine wrinkles, acne, skin laxity, and texture. The amount of retinol used was 0.075 percent, and the amount of salicylic acid, 2 percent. It was unclear whether the retinal or salicylic acid caused the changes.

Also, in order to be effective, the product should be manufactured under low-light conditions. Unfortunately, you can't tell by the label if a product has been produced to ensure its stability. But there are other things you can do to make sure you get an effective product. When shopping for and using OTC retinol products, Dr. Baumann advises consumers to:

- Look for products that are packaged in lightproof containers, such as aluminum tubes.
- Buy reputable brands. Ask your dermatologist for help.
- Look for products that contain 0.04 to 0.08 percent retinol.
- Apply retinol products at night to help maintain their stability.

Other Ingredients in Cosmeceuticals

Alpha Lipoic Acid. This antioxidant, which was discovered in 1951, is found in every cell in the body. Along with being a powerful free-radical fighter in its own right, it is also believed to increase the abilities of other antioxidants as well.

Limited studies have suggested that creams and lotions that contain alpha lipoic acid may help reduce fine lines and wrinkles and reduce puffiness under the eyes. More research is needed to substantiate these benefits.

Coenzyme Q10. Coenzyme Q10, a naturally occurring antioxidant found in the skin, is one of the newest ingredients being added to skin-care products. Several studies have made claims that have paved its way into the marketplace.

Just before the new millennium began, researchers in Germany released the results of a study in which they found that the use of topical coenzyme Q10 (ubiquinone; CoQ10), a naturally occurring and powerful antioxidant that is found in the skin, can help prevent many of the damaging effects of exposure to the sun. The investigators found that topical CoQ10 penetrates the top layer of skin, reduces wrinkle depth, and is effective against damage caused by ultraviolet A rays, especially the damage done to collagen and elastin. In another study conducted at a skin research center in Hamburg, Germany, investigators found that using a topical CoQ10 for six weeks daily reduced the wrinkle depth of crow's-feet by 27 percent, and after 10 weeks, by 43 percent.

It may still be too early to determine whether coenzyme Q10 is a significant player in the topical skin-care arena. Some doctors are very convinced; others are more cautious.

Ongoing studies may soon provide more answers. In the meantime, besides product cost, there are few downsides to its use.

Collagen. Collagen is a protein and a critical component in healthy skin. Natural collagen in the skin decreases at a rate of about 1 percent beginning in the third decade. It makes sense that you would want to find a way to prevent its loss, and it seems logical for manufacturers to add it to skin-care products. Unfortunately, when collagen is added to cosmetics, its only benefit is that it acts as a moisturizer. It will not have any effect on the collagen in your skin. Any manufacturer that claims the collagen in their product will increase the production, quantity, or quality of the collagen in your skin is not telling the truth. We know this because collagen molecules are too large to penetrate the skin to effect any change in the dermis, where collagen resides.

Although collagen is a decent moisturizer, it is also expensive. Other less costly ingredients can moisturize your skin just as well (see "What's in Your Moisturizer?" further in this chapter).

Copper. Creams that contain copper peptides were first developed for burn victims and for people who had diabetic wounds that would not heal. Now they are one of the newest additions to the skin-care market.

Dr. Baumann is an advocate of copper peptide, a relatively new addition to the anti-aging arena. "Copper peptide has been shown to stimulate collagen synthesis," she says, which makes it a critical helper in the war against aging. Results from several studies have shown that use of a copper peptide–containing cream significantly improved the appearance of fine lines and wrinkles, as well as increased skin thickness.

Participants were pleased with the results and there were no serious side effects.

When shopping for products that contain copper peptides, look for the words "GHK complex" or "copper peptide complex" on the ingredient panel.

Grape Seed Extract. Grape seed extract contains several powerful antioxidants known collectively as oligomeric proanthocyanidins (OPCs). Several studies done in Europe suggest that OPCs help prevent the breakdown of collagen and elastin in the skin, but these findings have not been proven. Some manufacturers have taken this information, however, and used it to make claims that grape seed extract is an important ingredient in their products. More research is needed before the validity of these claims can be determined.

Green Tea. Many studies have shown that green tea contains a powerful ingredient called epigallocatechin gallate (EGCG), an antioxidant that is effective in the fight against skin cancer. In particular, the application of EGCG to the skin of mice protected their skin from blistering and reddening when it was exposed to ultraviolet light. Preliminary experiments on human skin have shown that EGCG helps prevent inflammation and slows the development of skin cancer.

Whether the addition of EGCG to cosmetics will significantly benefit the skin is still in question. Again, further studies are needed to substantiate these findings.

Keratin. Keratin is a protein that is found in the epidermis. It is often added to moisturizers because it retains water, but it has no effect on the keratin in your skin. The keratin found in some moisturizers is derived from cow horns, boar bristles, or horse hair.

Kinetin. The chemical name for this substance is furfuryladenine, a plant enzyme that is being added to some lotions and creams to help soften the skin and reduce the appearance of fine lines and brown spots. Studies show that it increases moisture retention and slows the aging process in plants, while two studies at the University of California (Irvine) report that it also reduces aging in human cells. Some experts believe this very expensive additive does nothing for the skin and is best avoided. Further studies should clarify its role in skin rejuvenation.

Placenta. The placenta is the organ that provides nutrition to the fetus in the womb. When added to cosmetics, it is usually derived from cows. Claims that the addition of placenta extract (which is a mixture of proteins) will improve blood circulation and stimulate skin metabolism have no basis in fact. It has no effect on wrinkles and it is an expensive ingredient you can do without.

Vitamin C. When it comes to vitamin C, is it best in your orange juice but wasted on your face? Doctors don't agree about the value of applying products to the skin that contain vitamin C. One recent U.S. study has shown that a 10 percent ascorbic acid (vitamin C) cream can speed up resolution of the redness that occurs with laser resurfacing. In a recent study conducted in France, researchers showed that application of a 5 percent vitamin C cream to creases in the neck achieved significant improvement in wrinkles after six months of treatment.

The concern about vitamin C, however, is that in order for creams and lotions that contain the vitamin to be effective, they must be able to penetrate the skin, and they must remain potent. Therefore, several criteria must be met:

- Because vitamin C molecules are large, we know they cannot penetrate the skin. However, based on a few studies, some believe that the L-ascorbic form can achieve this goal and that topical vitamin C products that contain this form are effective. Research continues to look for ways that topical vitamin C can enter the skin.

- The vitamin must remain potent. Unfortunately, vitamin C is unstable and becomes ineffective when it is exposed to light. Therefore, any product containing vitamin C should be manufactured under special lighting conditions, packaged in an opaque container, and be stored in a dark place, preferably in the refrigerator. (Naturally, you don't know how a product was manufactured.) If you leave the top off of the product, it may lose nearly all of its potency.

- For a product to be effective, vitamin C must be present in a concentration of at least 10 percent, as indicated in the study mentioned above. Ten percent ascorbic acid may also help with other skin problems as well. But it also can irritate the skin of some users.

While no significant side effects have been attributed to the use of topical vitamin C, like so many other products, the proven benefits need qualification with ongoing studies.

Vitamin E. For many years, people have used vitamin E oil on their skin to help relieve sunburn. Vitamin E penetrates the epidermis, and reportedly helps reduce the loss of moisture, which can help protect against dry skin. A small percentage of people experience skin irritation from topical vitamin E, so you should apply a small amount to your inner arm before you decide to put it elsewhere on your body, and especially on your face.

Dr. Baumann says that vitamin E, when used in a topical

product, is a "good preservative to increase the shelf life of the product, and it gives it emollient (moisturizing) properties." Beyond that, she says, there's no research to back up any other claims made about it when it comes to skin care.

THE STORY OF SOAP

Wondering whatever happened to the old advice "Wash your face with soap and water"? Well, it's been updated.

Soaps are supposed to help remove oil and dirt from the skin. If you want to use soap to wash your body, that's one thing. But when it comes to washing your face, you need something that is nonirritating and mild while being effective. Today we have products other than soaps that help us do that, including exfoliants and cleansers.

True soaps have several problems. One, they contain fats (e.g., lard, tallow, tallowate) that can block your pores. Two, they can have a negative effect on the good bacteria that live on the surface of your skin. Three, most of them have a pH value between 9 and 10, while that of healthy skin is between 5.6 and 5.8. If you wanted to find the pH value on a given soap, you would have to contact the manufacturer, because that information isn't available on the packaging. Using a soap with a high pH will leave your face irritated and dry.

So forget the old advice. There are many soap-free cleansers on the market.

WHAT'S IN YOUR CLEANSER?

The number of facial cleansers on the market today can make your head spin. When you look at the ingredient panel, it can make your head spin even more. Which ingredients are the most beneficial? Which ones can irritate your skin? How do you know the difference between the two?

One thing is for certain: you can't always count on the advertising that markets these products. Many manufacturers will try to sell you ingredients that do little or nothing for your skin. When shopping for a cleanser, remember this: although you want an effective product, you don't need to spend a lot of money on fancy ingredients. Cleansers are only on your face for less than one minute per application. If you want to spend more money, save it for your moisturizer, which stays on your face all day. You need to be a savvy consumer.

No one product is best for everyone. Everyone has different skin types and sensitivities. But there are some general ingredients you can feel relatively sure will be good to your skin. Below is a list to consider. Also when shopping for a cleanser, keep in mind the ingredients we discussed earlier in this chapter. Some of them may be found in cleansing products.

- Purified water: This should be the first ingredient on the product's list. You want a good source of hydration and a purified water base in your cleanser.
- Sodium cocoyl isothionate: This cleansing agent comes from coconuts and is very mild.
- Alpha hydroxy acids (AHA): You learned about these earlier. Alpha hydroxy acids help exfoliate (remove) the top layer of skin cells and leave your skin cleaner and smoother.
- Propylene glycol: It helps to retain moisture and is oil-free.

- Salicylic acid: This beta hydroxy acid helps reduce skin redness, prevents acne, and provides a mild chemical peel. Because it may dry your skin if it is used every day, you may want to use it three times a week, alternating with other products in between.
- Chamomile: Since ancient times, this herbal ingredient has been used for its ability to soothe the skin. It's not essential, but it's a nice ingredient to have in your cleanser.

As a general rule of thumb, if you tend to get pimples, blackheads, or eczema, cleansers that contain salicylic acid or benzoyl peroxide are helpful.

Here are some of the ingredients you want to avoid when buying facial cleansers:

- Diethanolamine, ethanolamine, monoethanolamine, and triethanolamine. They may be listed as ETA on the label. These chemicals may cause liver cancer.
- Ammonium lauryl: This ingredient, as well as any other with the word "ammonium" attached to it (e.g., ammonium laureth sulfate, ammonium lauryl sulfate) can dry and irritate the skin.
- Alcohol: This ingredient can be very irritating and drying to the skin.
- Detergents: These can appear in products under many different names, including, but not limited to, cocamide DEA, sodium C14-16 olefin sulfate, sodium dodecyl sulfate, and TEA lauryl sulfate. Detergents can dry and irritate the skin.
- Mineral oil: This substance can clog your pores and leave your skin feeling slick and greasy.

One last thing before we move on to moisturizers. When you wash your face, use warm water: not hot, not cold. When you shock the delicate blood vessels in your face with hot or cold water, they can break. Extremes in water temperature can also irritate your skin. The steps for cleansing your face are:

- Place a small amount of cleanser on your fingertips.
- Gently rub the cleanser over your face for about 30 seconds.
- Remove the cleanser by splashing warm running water over your face several times until it feels as though the cleanser is gone.
- Use a clean towel to pat your face slightly, but keep your face damp. Moisturizer (one that contains sunscreen) should be applied to damp skin.

WHAT'S IN YOUR MOISTURIZER?

When choosing a moisturizer, you need to consider your skin type. Generally, if you have an oily complexion, tend to get pimples or blocked pores, or have acne or rosacea, choose a moisturizer that is oil-free. Such moisturizers typically contain glycolic acid or another alpha hydroxy acid, glycerin, salicylic acid, or propylene glycol. These ingredients help seal in water without oil.

If you aren't prone to skin breakouts, then you can choose among the many moisturizers on the market. If you have dry, sensitive skin, consider a cream or emollient that will be more hydrating for you.

The recommended ingredients to look for in a moisturizer

are listed below. Naturally, you don't need a product that contains all of them.

- Glycerin: A humectant (substance that holds moisture in the skin) that also helps loosen dry skin cells. Very effective against dry skin.
- Sodium hyaluronate: This ingredient retains moisture in the skin and is also an excellent lubricant.
- Vegetal squalane: A derivative of olives, this ingredient contains a high concentration of fats (oils) that help moisturize the skin.
- Urea: This natural moisturizer helps keep water on the skin's surface. It is very effective against dry skin.
- Rosewater: This mild moisturizer has been used for thousands of years. It helps all types of skin.
- Jojoba oil: The plant from which this oil is derived can withstand temperatures of more than 110 degrees and scarce rainfall. Those qualities make it an excellent ingredient to keep moisture locked into the skin.
- Vitamin E: As discussed earlier, this is a good moisturizer.

Avoid the following ingredients when purchasing a moisturizer:

- Fragrances: A moisturizer should moisturize. Period. There is no benefit for you if it contains fragrances or perfumes, which may irritate your skin.
- Acetylated lanolin: Derived from sheep's wool, this ingredient clogs your pores and may cause your skin to break out in a rash.
- Cocoa butter: True, it can moisturize your skin, but it

can also irritate it. There are so many other ingredients that moisturize, that it's best to avoid this one.

- Tallow: Plain and simple, this is animal fat. Avoid this pore-clogging ingredient.

When applying moisturizer, always put it on while your skin is damp. This prevents the evaporation of water that is still on your skin. It also helps you apply the moisturizer more evenly and allows for better absorption.

PUTTING IT ALL TOGETHER: SIMPLE STEPS TO SKIN CARE

If you're like most women, you have a busy schedule, and you don't have a lot of time to devote to your face. Therefore, you want to maximize the time you *do* spend by focusing on providing the best care possible.

A basic skin-care routine should include the following steps, but please talk to your dermatologist about your specific needs:

- Cleanse your face twice daily: in the morning and before bed at night.

- Apply moisturizer to your still-moist face. Your morning moisturizer should contain a broad-spectrum (containing ingredients that block both UVA and UVB rays) sunscreen with an SPF of at least 15. You may or may not choose a morning moisturizer that also contains a wrinkle-reducing ingredient such as alpha hydroxy acid. However, overuse of AHAs can irritate the skin, so you may want to reserve this ingredient for your nighttime moisturizer. Your nighttime moisturizer should contain ingredients such as an alpha hydroxy or beta hydroxy, vitamin A, or other products, depending on your skin type and individual needs (e.g., rough dry skin, oily skin, rosacea, acne). Remember: products that contain vitamin A should be applied at night to maintain their stability (see "Vitamin A" on page 175).

• Apply sunscreen (if your moisturizer doesn't contain it) in the morning after your moisturizer has dried. You will still need to apply a sunscreen over your moisturizer throughout the day if you are exposed to the sun.

SOME FINAL WORDS: BUYER BEWARE

Vitamin and other nutritional supplements, herbs, and cosmetics (for the most part) are not drugs, are not strictly regulated by the Food and Drug Administration (FDA), and therefore do not have FDA approval. Although these products are tested for safety, they are not subject to mandatory review by the FDA, and their effectiveness does not have to be proven. Many of the claims made by cosmetic manufacturers are very alluring and hold out hope to people who may be looking for a silver bullet. In fact, many claims about cosmetics cannot be validated scientifically. They are worded carefully to suggest that users will gain some therapeutic advantages from the product, but because these benefits have not been analyzed and approved by the FDA, the producers are prohibited from making definitive claims.

Therefore, it's a matter of **buyer beware.** Unfortunately, along with the uncertainty about the effectiveness of these products, many cosmetics are very expensive, and you can waste a lot of money and time experimenting with different ones. Your best bet: learn all you can about the effectiveness of the ingredients that are being touted in the advertisements of any cosmetic product. That means reading the results of studies that have been done (the Internet can be a big help here; be suspicious of any bias in research that has been conducted by the manufacturer of the product), talk to your doctor, and ask other people about their experiences with the ingredients and products in question. And if the claims sound too good to be true, it's probably because they are.

QUESTIONS AND ANSWERS

I used a product that contains vitamin A on my face and my face got red and irritated. A friend told me that that was a sign the product was working. Is she right?

To some extent, irritation is an expected side effect of vitamin A products, which is why Dr. Sengelmann has her patients begin by applying vitamin A products every other to every third day. Over time, your skin will better tolerate more frequent use of the product. If, however, you don't begin to tolerate it better, talk to your doctor.

If you are using a prescription vitamin A product, you can ask your doctor if there is a less-irritating product you can use. There's no guarantee, however, that this less-irritating brand will not cause you a problem as well. If you are using an over-the-counter brand, which contains a lower percentage of the vitamin A derivatives than prescription brands, the fact that you reacted to the product may be an indication that your skin is too sensitive to use products that contain vitamin A, or it may be a sign of allergy to another ingredient in the product. Talk to your dermatologist.

Should I get moisturizers that contain collagen or elastin? Will they reduce or eliminate my wrinkles and fine lines?

Moisturizers, or any other skin product, that contain collagen or elastin will often claim that these ingredients will do wondrous things for your skin. They usually mention the fact that collagen and elastin, in particular, are present in the second layer of skin (the dermis) and are critical for healthy, wrinkle-free skin. And this is true. So the manufacturers want you to believe that using their products will help in "replacing essential elements that your skin has lost," and other similar claims. These statements are not true.

In reality, the molecules of these ingredients are too large to penetrate the dermis, where they are needed. The only way collagen is going to help your wrinkles is if you inject it, or if you stimulate its development with chemical peels or laser treatments. Otherwise, it's just a moisturizer.

Although these moisturizers will help hold in moisture for a short amount of time, they cannot eliminate wrinkles or fine lines. And when you look at the products that contain collagen and elastin, you'll realize that you're going to be paying a pretty high price for that moisturizer when a lower-priced or even generic brand will do just as well.

Remember: no moisturizer will eliminate wrinkles. All moisturizers do is hydrate dry skin, thus making it look better.

A friend told me to try a moisturizer that contains placenta, because it will improve blood circulation to my face and help remove wrinkles. Is she right?

The placenta is the organ that transports nutrients to the fetus in humans and all other mammals. Cow placentas are the most common source of the placental extract in products like the one your friend is suggesting. Any claim that a cream that contains a placenta extract, which is a combination of proteins, will eliminate wrinkles is not based on any scientific evidence.

My dermatologist recommended that I use an alpha hydroxy acid cream. What is alpha hydroxy acid?

Alpha hydroxy acids (AHAs) are naturally occurring compounds that can help keep the skin moist by trapping water within it. They can also help unplug pores, through the exfoliation (shedding of dead skin cells) of your outer layer of skin, and, with regular long-term use, can stimulate the production of elastin in your dermis.

But there is such a thing as too much of a good thing. Use AHA lotions and creams as instructed by your dermatologist. Overuse can cause your skin to get itchy and red. If this happens, you can switch to a beta hydroxy acid (BHA), such as salicylic acid, which is somewhat milder and less likely to cause irritation.

Isn't it true that the more expensive moisturizers are better for the skin than a less expensive or generic brand?

Not at all. When shopping for a moisturizer, the first thing you should be looking at is the ingredient list, not the price tag. Look for beneficial ingredients, like glycerin, sodium hyaluronate, vitamin E, and vegetal squalane. Avoid expensive come-ons in product ingredients like collagen and keratin or additives that may be irritating, such as perfumes or cocoa butter. The point of buying a moisturizer is to moisturize your face, not spend a small fortune.

I read the ingredient panel on my facial cleanser and although the product contains alpha hydroxy acid, it doesn't say what the concentration and pH are. Why not?

The Food and Drug Administration does not require manufacturers to reveal the concentration of AHAs in a product, nor the pH. However, you can contact the manufacturer and ask for that information. There should be some contact information on the product's packaging. You may also try to find the manufacturer on the Internet and pose your question there.

What's the difference between a "facial" soap and a "body" soap? Is there any kind of soap that's best for cleansing the face?

Facial and body bars are the same, although you may have to pay more for the facial variety. Soaps that claim to be "natural" often contain tallow, tallowate, or sodium laureate as the main ingredient, and are no better or milder than many other soaps. Deodorant soaps should never be used on the face because their pH value can cause irritation. When it comes to cleaning your face, nonsoap cleansers are best. Even though mild cleansers don't "soap up" with lather, they are still doing their job—removing oil, makeup, and dirt.

Just a few words about shower gels. Some people think these products are better for their skin than bar soap. In reality, most shower gels contain a lot of fragrances that can irritate the skin and cause skin allergies. Some of the gels also come with scrubbers, which can promote bacterial growth. And shower gels are usually more expensive than soap. All in all, shower gels are not a good bet for your skin, and especially not for your face.

How effective are oxygen facials for keeping facial skin young looking? A local spa offers them, and I've been wanting to try one.

Blowing oxygen onto your skin has absolutely no benefits, except for the wallet of the person doing the treatment. Oxygen does not penetrate the skin; your skin gets its oxygen supply through the bloodstream via the lungs. Don't waste your time and money.

GLOSSARY

Ablation. Removal of thin layers of tissue. Thus, non-ablation laser techniques are processes that do not remove those layers (see "non-ablative laser").

Alpha hydroxy acids (AHAs). Naturally occurring substances that are derived from fruits (e.g., apples, grapes, and citrus), sugarcane, and sour milk. They are used as an exfoliant, a substance that helps remove the dead layer of skin.

Alpha lipoic acid. An antioxidant that reportedly helps in the fight against lines and wrinkles.

Antioxidant. A compound that fights free radicals, molecules that contribute to the aging process. Common antioxidants include vitamins A, C, and E; the minerals selenium and zinc; and the substance coenzyme Q10.

Arachidonic acid. A type of essential fatty acid that is involved in causing inflammation of the skin. It can be converted by vitamin C into less-harmful substances.

Autologous fat injection. Process in which fat that has been harvested from one area of the body is injected into another. Fat injections are used as wrinkle fillers.

Basal cell. A type of cell that is found at the bottom of the epidermis.

Beta hydroxy acids (BHAs). A family of chemicals that are used as exfoliants and that cause less irritation than the alpha hydroxy acids (AHAs).

Blepharospasm. A type of dystonia characterized by uncontrolled twitching or spasm of the muscles around the eye.

Botox. A toxin that is derived from the bacterium *Clostridium botulinum*. Botox is injected into the muscles in the forehead and around the eyes to relax the muscles and help eliminate muscle-driven wrinkles. It is also used to relax the muscles in various medical conditions, such as migraine, strabismus, and lower back pain.

Chemical peel. The application of an acid formulation to the skin that helps remove fine lines and wrinkles and reduce blotchiness.

Cleanser. A substance or formula that removes dirt, dead skin cells, oils, and makeup from the skin.

Collagen. A protein found in the dermis that is essential for maintaining the structure of the skin.

Corrugator supercilii: Muscle in the forehead area that causes your eyebrows to lower. It is also involved in the formation of vertical furrows between the brows.

Cosmeceuticals. Topical cosmetic products that reportedly have medicinal properties to enhance the beauty and health of the skin.

Crow's-feet. The lines that radiate from the outer corners of the eyes. They are the result of muscle contractions, such as squinting and aging.

Depressor supercilii. Muscle in the forehead area that causes the eyebrows to lower.

Dermabrasion. A procedure that involves the use of a high-speed sanding device that helps smooth the skin and remove fine lines, wrinkles, and acne scars.

Dermis. The layer of skin that lies below the top layer (epidermis). The dermis is inhabited by collagen, elastin, blood vessels, nerves, sweat glands, oil glands, and hair follicles, and is also where wrinkles are born.

Dynamic wrinkles. Lines and creases in the skin that are caused by facial expressions such as smiling, frowning, squinting, and laughing, which contract the underlying muscles.

Dystonia. A condition characterized by abnormal, involuntary, and sustained muscle contractions that result in repetitive movements or abnormal postures. Examples include cervical dystonia, blepharospasm, and hemifacial spasm.

Elasticity. The ability of skin, tissue, or muscle to return to its original shape.

Elastin. A type of tissue found in the dermis that helps the skin maintain its elasticity and resilience.

Epidermis. The outer layer of skin.

Estrogen. A female hormone that plays a role in skin health. Low levels of the hormone can cause dry skin and contribute to wrinkling.

Exfoliant. A substance that helps remove the outer layer of dry, dead skin cells to reveal the smoother layer beneath it.

Free radicals. Molecules that can cause damage to cells and contribute to the aging process.

Frontalis. Muscle in the forehead that helps you raise your eyebrows; it is also responsible for the horizontal wrinkles that can form across your forehead.

Glabellar lines. The vertical wrinkles in the forehead that lie between the eyebrows.

Glycolic acid. A type of alpha hydroxy acid that is derived from sugarcane. It is used for light chemical peels.

Herpes. A viral disease characterized by blisters on the skin and the mucous membranes.

Humectant. A substance that helps retain moisture in the skin.

Hydroquinones. Substances that are used to lighten or "bleach" the skin.

Hyperpigmentation: Darkening of the skin.

Hypopigmentation. Lightening of the skin.

Keratin. A type of protein that is part of the outer layer of the skin.

Keratinocyte. A cell found in the epidermis that produces keratin.

Laser resurfacing. A process in which the layers of the skin are vaporized with a laser beam for the purpose of eliminating wrinkles and other skin abnormalities.

Laugh lines. The lines or creases that appear at the corners of your nose and descend to the outer corners of your mouth.

Lidocaine. A local anesthetic that can be injected or applied as a cream to reduce pain. It is often applied to the skin before various cosmetic procedures, such as Botox injections and collagen injections.

Marionette lines. The wrinkles that extend from the corners of the mouth toward the jaw.

Melanin. The pigment in the skin that is responsible for skin color.

Mineral oil. A derivative of petroleum that is used in many moisturizers.

Nasolabial folds. Also known as laugh or smile lines, they are the creases that extend from the corners of the nose to the corners of the mouth.

Non-ablative laser. A laser technique that eliminates wrinkles without damaging the skin.

Orbicularis oculi: The muscle that closes the eye; it is also involved in the formation of crow's-feet.

Phenol. A chemical that is used to achieve a deep chemical peel for the purpose of eliminating wrinkles and acne scars.

Photo aging. The response of the skin to a lifetime of ultraviolet rays. Reactions include the formation of lines and wrinkles, loss of skin elasticity, brown spots, changes in pigmentation, and broken blood vessels.

Procurus. Muscle involved in the formation of frown lines that appear between the eyebrows.

Retin-A. The brand name of a prescription medication that contains tretinoin, a derivative of vitamin A. Retin-A is used to treat sun-damaged skin and acne.

Salicylic acid. A cousin to aspirin, this substance has anti-inflammatory capabilities. It also has been found to be helpful in the treatment of aging skin.

Self-tanners. Products that contain a water-soluble, nontoxic dye (dihydroxyacetone, or DHA) that gives the skin a tanned look. They may or may not contain a sunscreen.

Strabismus. Also known as cross-eye, it is a condition characterized by an inability to focus both eyes.

Stratum corneum. The uppermost layer of the epidermis. It is sometimes referred to as the horny layer because it consists of dead skin cells.

Subcutis. The layer of fat that lies beneath the dermis.

Sun-protection factor (SPF). A number used to indicate how effective a sunscreen is in preventing sunburn.

Sunscreen. A product that protects the skin against ultraviolet radiation by absorbing the rays.

Surfactants. Natural or synthetic substances that break up grease, oil, and water so they can better cleanse the skin.

Tretinoin. A derivative of vitamin A, and the active ingredient in Retin-A.

Trichloracetic acid (TCA). A chemical used during a medium chemical peel to treat wrinkles, acne scars, and sun-damaged skin.

Ultraviolet (UV) light. Invisible, high-energy light that comes from the sun, of which two types, UVA and UVB, can cause damage to the skin.

Vitamin A. An antioxidant that benefits the skin when taken orally and applied topically.

APPENDIX

Resources for Information About Cosmetic Uses of Botox and Other Cosmetic Procedures

American Academy of Dermatology
930 E. Woodfield Rd.
Schaumburg, IL 60173-6016
888-462-DERM (3376)
www.aad.org

American Academy of Facial Plastic and Reconstructive Surgery
1110 Vermont Avenue, NW, Suite 220
Washington, DC 20005-3522
202-842-4500
www.facial-plastic-surgery.org

American Society for Aesthetic Plastic Surgery, Inc.
444 East Algonquin Road, Suite 110
Arlington Heights, IL 60005
847-228-9274
www.surgery.org

American Society for Dermatologic Surgery
930 N. Meacham Road
Schaumburg, IL 60168-4014
Information Service: 800-441-2737
www.asds-net.org

American Society of Ophthalmic Plastic and Reconstructive
Surgery
1133 West Morse Blvd, #201
Winter Park, FL 32789
407-647-8839

Resources for Medical Uses of Botox

American Academy of Neurology
1080 Montreal Avenue
St. Paul, MN 55116
651-695-1940
www.aan.com

American Chronic Pain Association (ACPA)
P.O. Box 850
Rocklin, CA 95677-0850
916-632-0922
www.theacpa.org

American Council for Headache Education
19 Mantua Road
Mt. Royal, NJ 08061
856-423-0258
www.achenet.org

Benign Essential Blepharospasm Research Foundation, Inc.
637 North 7th Street, Suite 102
P.O. Box 12468

Beaumont, TX 77726-2468
409-832-0788
www.blepharospasm.org

Fibromyalgia Network
P.O. Box 31750
Tucson, AZ 85751-1750
800-853-2929
Contact: Ms. Kristin Thorson

Hemifacial Spasm Association
An on-line support group
www.hfs-assn.org/index.htm

National Fibromyalgia Association
2238 N. Glassell Street, Suite D
Orange, CA 92865
714-921-0150
www.nfa.org

National Headache Foundation
888-NHF-5552
www.headaches.org

National Institute of Neurological Disorders & Stroke
800-352-9424
www.ninds.nih/gov/

National Organization for Rare Disorders (NORD)
P.O. Box 8923
(100 Route 37)
New Fairfield, CT 06812-8923
800-999-NORD (6673)
www.rarediseases.org

National Spasmodic Torticollis Association
9920 Talbert Avenue, #233

Fountain Valley, CA 92708
800-HURTFUL

National Stroke Association
9707 E. Easter Lane
Englewood, CO 80112
800-STROKES
www.stroke.org

Resources for Cosmetic Products and Supplements
Cosmetics
www.skinstore.com
www.cosmeticmall.com
www.drugstore.com
www.beautydoor.com
www.gloss.com
www.cosmeticconnection.com provides a list of more than
100 cosmetic companies, their telephone numbers (many
toll-free), and websites

Supplements
www.iherb.com/vitamineral.html
www.vitamins.com
www.discount-vitamins-herbs.net
www.basicvitamins.com
www.vitaminworld.com

INDEX